"Readers of all ages can relate to Tim's story of trying to find one's way in life ... Romance, Riches, and Restrooms gives us a glimpse into the solitary struggles of a person whose life is under siege by irritable bowel syndrome. At times laugh-out-loud funny and at times poignantly heartbreaking, Tim's book educates us all as to the realities of IBS and in doing so will hopefully make it easier for other sufferers to access the help they need."

—Barbara Bradley Bolen, Clinical Psychologist, Author of *Breaking the Bonds of Irritable Bowel Syndrome*

"Tim's true-to-life recount of learning what ails his bowel is so easily identifiable for many IBS sufferers; however, Tim didn't write his memoir for just IBS sufferers. His aim was to inform everyone that there are quality of life issues that IBS sufferers face each and every day. He engagingly plastered his very personal story on the pages of his book to raise awareness about this illness."

—Jeffrey Roberts, President and Founder, Irritable Bowl Syndrome Self-Help and Support Group

"From the start of Tim's book I was struck by Tim Phelan's easily readable writing style. I recommend this book as a good informative read, which will make you laugh and empathize with the character ... It also offers an insight into various therapies and hope that one might offer if not a cure, a way forward to live with irritable bowel syndrome."

—Neil Davey, *Gut Reaction* (IBS Network quarterly journal)

"Romance, Riches, and Restrooms *is a very well-written, funny, and intelligent book that anyone with IBS will identify with. I would highly recommend it to all IBS sufferers. And if I had the power I would make all the loved ones of IBSers read it as well, as it is a fantastic explanation of how IBS can slowly take control of almost all aspects of your life, however successful or intelligent or confident you are.*"

—Sophie Lee, Founder of IBS Tales Web site

"*Irritable bowel syndrome is no laughing matter. At least, it wasn't until Tim Phelan came along. Along with more than 50 million other Americans, Tim suffers from IBS. But unlike most of those others, he's been able to mine some humor from his condition. The result is the book* Romance, Riches, and Restrooms: A Cautionary Tale of Ambitious Dreams and Irritable Bowels."

—Nina Sax, Gastroenterologist and Co-host of "The Health Show"

"*By discussing his IBS in an honest, self-deprecating, and humorous way, Tim has provided a valuable service for the millions who suffer in silence.*"

—Brent Ridge, Host of "The Visiting Hour" (Martha Stewart Living Channel)

"I've always said that all men and all women suffer equally under the tyranny of their bowels. But Phelan's entertaining book has taught me a very important lesson: some people clearly suffer a lot more than others."

—**Dave Praeger, Author of** ***Poop Culture: How America is Shaped by Its Grossest National Product***

"Romance, Riches, and Restrooms is an exceptionally vivid story ... Phelan makes his readers laugh, cry, reflect, and squirm like they've never squirmed before."

—**Sean Michael Flynn, Author of** ***Land of the Radioactive Midnight Sun: A Cheechako's First Year in Alaska***

"Romance, Riches, and Restrooms is one of the more entertaining, enlightening, and courageous memoirs ... The author opens up a new world in occasionally humorous, and more often moving, fashion."

—**Willaim Kerns, Entertainment Editor,** ***Lubbock Avalanche-Journal***

ROMANCE, RICHES, AND RESTROOMS

ROMANCE, RICHES, AND RESTROOMS

A CAUTIONARY TALE OF AMBITIOUS DREAMS AND IRRITABLE BOWELS

Tim Phelan

iUniverse Star
New York Lincoln Shanghai

ROMANCE, RICHES, AND RESTROOMS
A CAUTIONARY TALE OF AMBITIOUS DREAMS AND IRRITABLE BOWELS

iUniverse Star
an iUniverse, Inc. imprint

iUniverse books may be ordered through booksellers or by contacting:

iUniverse
2021 Pine Lake Road, Suite 100
Lincoln, NE 68512
www.iuniverse.com
1-800-Authors (1-800-288-4677)

Because of the dynamic nature of the Internet, any Web addresses or links contained in this book may have changed since publication and may no longer be valid.

The views expressed in this work are solely those of the author and do not necessarily reflect the views of the publisher, and the publisher hereby disclaims any responsibility for them.

ISBN: 978-1-58348-018-2 (pbk)
ISBN: 978-0-595-88906-8 (ebk)

Printed in the United States of America

Contents

Coming Clean

The events recounted in this memoir took place over seventeen years. In the interest of readability, I have occasionally altered the chronology and changed some events and characters into composites of different events or persons. Many (but certainly not all) of the names and identifying characteristics have been changed in an effort to protect people's privacy.

For reasons I still can't completely comprehend, and will likely live to regret, I have chosen to use my real name.

Prologue

Stacey was stunned. Of course, I'd seen it all before. The topic usually cropped up during the first date, sometimes the second. They all reacted the same way.

"Let me get this straight," she said. "You've never been to France?"

"No."

"Never?" she asked.

"Not even once."

"And you *majored* in French?"

"*Oui, c'est vrais.*"

"But you *have* been overseas, right? You just never made it to France?"

"Uh … no."

"How is that possible?"

I shrugged. "I guess it was just never the right time."

It was a lame, silly explanation. It also wasn't true.

I didn't want to deceive her, but the truth was a long, complicated story. Too revealing for first-date give-and-take. She might understand why I hadn't yet explored the world … or she might not. I didn't plan on finding out. I enjoyed her company, but I already suspected that another date was not in the cards. She seemed a little too adventurous.

"What a waste." She wasn't angry—more like disgusted. "Do you have any idea what you're missing?"

Now that was a stupid question. If I'd never been there, how could I?

If Stacey had any idea how much more I was missing in my life, she'd be horrified.

"Hey, it's not a total loss," I said. "At least I live in a city with great international food, right? I mean that's got to be worth *something.*"

Why step on a plane when I could taste some of the world's best food right in San Francisco? Downtown, near Union Square, Boulevard, Farallon, and Postrio served some of the city's most celebrated—but pricey—cuisine. The city was filled with diverse ethnic neighborhoods offering reasonably priced, regional culinary delights. For Italian there was North Beach. For Mexican you went down to the Mission District. In the mood for Chinese? We had our own Chinatown. Forget Paris.

"Good point," she conceded. "If you had to eat the rest of your meals at only one restaurant, which one would you pick?"

"How can I possibly answer that before I taste my enchiladas?" I asked.

It didn't seem like the right time to disclose that even though I'd lived there for the better part of a decade, I seldom ventured out to explore other neighborhoods in San Francisco. In fact, I never left my safe little universe in the Marina District unless I had to. Why risk it? Consequently I had made myself a full-fledged regular at a handful of neighborhood eateries on Chestnut Street. None were more than six or seven blocks from my apartment.

Here at Café Marimba, the atmosphere was funky, and the margaritas strong. This casually hip Mexican joint was the centerpiece of my first-date ritual. I wasn't much for surprises. When I found something that worked, I tended to stick with it. The only risk here was the waiter blowing my cover. This was my third first date that week.

Stacey couldn't let it go. "But you do want to see the world, don't you? I mean, someday?"

I looked up from my margarita. "Of course I want to. And someday, yes, I will."

That part was true. I had dreamed of international travel for years. In fact, that was a big reason I decided to study French in the first place. Most of my classmates followed the well-beaten path from college to commercial banking. Not me.

Like my banking-bound buddies, I majored in economics. But I also pursued French as a second major. The details of my plan were a bit fuzzy, but I would one day enjoy a wildly successful career in international business.

In truth, I didn't even know what such a career entailed. But traveling the world and making a lucrative living sounded so alluring. Not to mention the women. Of course, with my glamorous lifestyle I would attract all sorts of beautiful, sophisticated women. Eventually I would meet my future wife and start a family. But I'd have plenty of time for that. I was in no particular rush.

So how had I ended up here, more than a decade after college, unmarried and an overseas virgin with a passport still waiting for its first stamp?

The story began thirteen years earlier—ironically with one surprisingly powerful cup of French Roast coffee. From that moment on, my life would never be the same.

Follow the Leaders

It was 1988. Diploma in hand and poised for greatness, I waited for my coronation. Somewhere beyond the campus of Washington and Lee University, a great, exciting world was just waiting for me.

I couldn't wait to see Paris and the south of France, too. Surely the French would be impressed with my near-fluency in their native tongue. In due time, I would make my way to London, Rome, and the rest of Europe before jetting off to Australia and South America. I'd heard great things about Carnival.

Yes, I was ready to conquer the world.

But first I was headed to New Jersey. This seemingly curious beginning to my ambitious global conquest actually fit right into my plan. Four years earlier, I had graduated from Lawrenceville, a private boarding school near Princeton. Now I was back as a member of the faculty.

In a place where not much ever seemed to change, a *lot* had changed. Most notably this once all-male institution was now coed—too late, as it turned out, to reverse the damage caused by only occasional interaction with women during the four years leading up to my theoretical sexual peak. And after thirty-five years, the school now had a new headmaster at the helm. His name was Si Bunting.

As a rule, headmasters need to be scholars, disciplinarians, chief executives, and fund-raisers, too. As a result, they tend to be intimidating figures. Si not only fit the mold, but also took the intimidation factor to a whole new level.

Standing well over six feet tall, he had a fit, chiseled frame and a deep, booming voice. Headmasters aren't the kind of people you'd expect to sport tattoos, but Si was an exception. His tattoo was *not* from his combat tour with the U.S. Army in Vietnam—where, incidentally, he also picked up a Bronze Star—but from an earlier, post-high-school stint in the Marines. Covering most of his forearm, the sprawling ink job, visible to faculty and students alike as the headmaster ran through campus training for his marathons, sent a clear message: *Don't even* think *about messing with me.* As for academic credentials, he was a Rhodes Scholar. This guy was the real thing: a tough, disciplined leader who expected loyalty. You didn't have to always agree with him, but you crossed him at your own peril.

Getting the job meant beating out fifteen other alumni candidates and earning Si's stamp of approval. When I got the job, I was told I had made a great first impression on Si. That was nice to hear but not that surprising. In fact, I would have been shocked if I hadn't.

You see, making a great impression had always been my thing.

Like Si, I had done a few tours of duty myself—first in Cub Scouts, then in Boy Scouts, picking up a few of my own stars on the way. As best I could tell, all that Scout talk about being trustworthy, loyal, helpful, friendly, courteous, kind, and—what were the rest of them?—must have stuck to me, forming a halo above my head. Sure, I had one hell of a mischievous side, but to my surprise, nobody ever noticed … not at first, anyway.

Growing up, I was the well-behaved, wholesome boy next door with the all-American looks and the charming smile. People trusted me, unlike the Duffy boys down the street, who, if you weren't careful, might steal your bike.

I didn't always understand the impression that I made, but I knew it opened a lot of doors for me. Most recently it was an asset that helped me get into Phi Kappa Sigma, arguably the most popular fraternity on the W&L campus. It also did wonders for me in the college dating arena. I didn't always have a girlfriend, but I never had any trouble finding a date. I suspect it even played a role in my making the lacrosse team in college, too.

But never had this ability impacted my life more than when I was fourteen; it saved the day and changed the direction of my life. Only five months after my parents and I first drove from New York to Lawrenceville in my father's 1973 green Mercedes, Mr. Gerstell, an English teacher, came to my room to deliver the news. "Tim, I'm sorry, but your father can no longer pay your tuition." I was ashamed.

This was devastating, but it wasn't the first abrupt detour of my life. My parents had divorced five years earlier. My father was a charismatic Irish Catholic who worked hard and played even harder. In the end, his vices and addictions ultimately brought his rags-to-riches success story violently crashing down on him … and all of us. One day we had live-in maids, country clubs, and a Mercedes. The next day my mother, brother, sister, and I piled into a beat-up Volvo station wagon and moved into a cramped one-bedroom apartment outside Manhattan.

It was a difficult, painful transition, but in hindsight, it was clearly for the best. My father's Mercedes was the only evidence of the luxurious lifestyle we had once briefly enjoyed. Sending me to a prestigious prep school was neither a priority nor a financial possibility. It was preposterous. But my dad had insisted that he was back on his financial feet again. He wanted to play the role of big spender. If nothing else, he had good intentions.

I mentally packed my bags and thought about how I would explain my swift return to my classmates back at Hastings High. Mr. Gerstell made a proposition: "Even though you've only been here a short while, you're well liked, you've worked hard, and your grades are good." He said that as long as I kept this up, I could stay put. How was this possible? Who would pay for me to stay there?

That was when I learned that Lawrenceville's alumni donated quite a bit of money to the school each year. Their contributions to the Annual Giving Fund helped students whose parents couldn't afford the tuition.

There I was, after college, back at Lawrenceville. It seemed fitting that as the assistant director of Annual Giving, I was now responsible for raising money to help out the next generation of financially challenged students. This was my opportunity to begin to repay Lawrenceville for all it had done for me. My motives were noble, but not entirely altruistic. The salary was modest—pennies compared to what my friends were making in banking. That was OK. My payoff would come later.

Malcolm Forbes, Michael Eisner, and pop singer Huey Lewis were just some of the school's high-profile graduates. There was also Ken Hakuta, aka Dr. Fad, the genius inventor who sold 240 million Wacky WallWalkers. And there were more. Lots more. The alumni directory was packed with thousands of men who, while if not household names, were serious movers and shakers who could do wonders for my professional future after I completed my two-year stint. Who knew—maybe Dr. Fad would need help penetrating the French marketplace.

I would rub elbows with these magnates. The possibilities were endless. In my mind, winning over these powerful men was going to be a layup. All I had to do was what I always did best: make a good impression.

◆   ◆   ◆

Three months later, at the University Club in midtown Manhattan, it was showtime. This was my chance to shine.

They trickled into the cavernous banquet hall one by one. All in all, 150 or so New York area alumni had taken time away from running the world to be there. They came to catch up with old classmates, network with new friends, and see what this new headmaster was all about. Cocktails were sipped, the crowd seated, and lunch served.

I knew enough to put the napkin on my lap. But damn, exactly what was I supposed to do with all those forks and spoons? And what was the deal with those bread plates? My new pin-striped suit helped me look as if I belonged, but after four years of fraternity living, it dawned on me that my business-etiquette skills were not quite ready for prime time. I had come here to make a good impression, not to call attention to myself with a glaring faux pas. So I decided to sit back and follow everybody else's lead.

The talk at our table turned to international monetary policy and trends in the currency market. I was generally familiar with the terms being tossed about from my economics classes, but the discussion was too fast-paced for me to process. Any attempt to add value to this conversation would have been laughable. I remembered somebody once saying that it was better to keep quiet and have people think you were an idiot than to open your mouth and remove all doubt.

From mixed green salad to cream of potato soup to prime rib, I saw to it that my mouth was always full, letting nothing on my plate go to waste. When a hulking slab of New York cheesecake was set down in front of me, I gave it the same treatment.

I hadn't yet made a good impression, but I hadn't made a bad one, either.

Then came the fateful question.

"Excuse me, sir. Would you care for some coffee?"

Now, except for the occasional cup during college for all-night cram sessions, I was not much of a coffee drinker. But I was ready to be an adult. The movers and shakers all took coffee. It seemed like a rite of passage. I badly wanted to fit in. Was I naive enough to think a cup of caffeine would put me on par with these accomplished men? I thought about the question again. *Coffee? Well, why not?*

I struggled with my first few sips. I'd forgotten that coffee was an acquired taste my palate did not immediately embrace. To avoid looking like the rookie I was, I did my best to suppress any reflexive facial contortions that would relay just how much I disliked the taste. With each new mouthful, my taste buds became marginally more accepting of the French Roast.

Unfortunately the same could not be said of my insides. Little did I know that with this seemingly arbitrary decision, I was lighting the fuse to the Molotov cocktail I had just created in my intestines. I was only halfway through the cup when I knew a trip to the toilet was imminent. *One more bite of cheesecake, and then it's straight to the men's room.*

I was caught completely off guard. Why didn't I see it coming? No sooner had I emptied the cup and stuffed another forkful of dessert into my mouth than I heard the unmistakable, commanding voice from the microphone at the podium: "Good afternoon. My name is Josiah Bunting. Thank you for joining us today …"

No. This can't be happening!

When I think back to that exact moment, I picture the expression on Wile E. Coyote's face, suspended in midair after running off the five-hundred-foot cliff, at the precise second he realizes that the immutable law of gravity is about to kick in. His fate will be sealed. There is nothing he can do about it. I didn't realize it at the time, but I had just taken my first step down a long, slippery slope.

The huge room fell silent. All eyes focused on the man at the microphone.

When I had gotten out of bed earlier that morning, I was dying to be in the inner circle, beneath the spotlight, impressing the hell out of my audience. Now here I was, at the main event. I even had a front-row seat, no more than six feet from where my boss had embarked on what I knew would be a one-hour speech. As they say, be careful what you wish for. Now that I was finally here, I desperately had to go.

Now what would I do? What *could* I do? From his position high atop the elevated speaker's podium, Si towered almost directly above me, appearing more intimidating than ever. He had just begun his speech. If I excused myself to use the men's room now, how would that make me look? Rude and unprofessional, I quickly concluded. What would the man who signed my paychecks think of me? As the low man on the totem pole in our office, I was more or less expendable. Even if Si wouldn't fire me over such a disruption, a serious reprimand seemed likely.

In a sea of confident and accomplished men, I was a self-conscious neophyte. This was nothing short of a moral dilemma. Bits and pieces of the Boy Scout oath came rushing back to me. A Scout should be loyal, obedient, and brave—three traits that my current predicament certainly required ... and that the headmaster no doubt expected. No problem there. But lastly a Scout should also be clean. My values were in conflict.

As I tried to listen to the content of his talk, his words were drowned out by the message coming from my gut.

"We have a crisis down here that demands immediate attention and cannot be ignored!" it seemed to be saying.

My mind quickly shot back, "Can't this wait for an hour?"

"Not likely," was the prompt response from below.

Now what?

How stupid! Why hadn't I gotten up and gone when I had the chance? *Arrrggggg!* I was a little rusty on my childhood Sunday school lessons, but I seemed to recall one of the deadly sins being gluttony. I'd never been devoutly religious, but I couldn't help but wonder if I was now being punished for the sin of eating that last bite of cheesecake.

I glanced around the room. No waiters refilling coffee cups. No bus-boys clearing plates. Nobody even flinching. The minutes crawled by.

Physically nothing prevented me from getting up and going to the men's room, but I'd always felt enormous pressure to abide by proper decorum. From my earliest childhood memory, I never wanted to stand out, make any waves, or call attention to myself. My biggest priority was to just fit in with everyone else.

If all the other kids wore Levi's jeans, then I didn't want to be the dork who showed up wearing the hideous Sears Tuffskins. Of course, I preferred to do well, but falling short of the norm was what terrified me. It would have been great to score 1,500 on my SATs, but if the average score was 1,100 ... well then, 1,100 would be just fine. *But please don't let me be the guy bringing up the rear with 850. Don't let me be the only person unable to endure lunch, coffee, and a one-hour speech without visiting the men's room. I sure as hell don't want to be the guy who causes a scene by running out before the speech is done.* Was that too much to ask?

It was only a matter of time. Surely somebody would eventually stand up and walk to the restroom. Somebody had to. We had all just eaten the same meal. It seemed statistically unlikely that I would be the only one in desperate need of relief.

As I had done before laying even a finger on my silverware or bread plate, I would wait to follow somebody else's lead. Let another man irreverently rise up and shatter the stillness, I figured. And if that first, brave soul wasn't pelted with sugar cubes, assaulted by disapproving glances, or taken to task by the headmaster ... well then, the coast would be clear for me, too. Yes, I would have to wait.

And wait ... and wait ... and wait.

The stillness intensified.

As I glanced over my shoulder toward the back of the room—and the only exit—I found three hundred eyes staring intently at the austere speaker above and behind me. I didn't get it. No doubt Si was a naturally powerful and engaging speaker, but he was the headmaster of a boarding school—not the pope. These people were absolutely transfixed. The movers and shakers were neither moving nor shaking. As far as I could tell, they weren't blinking or breathing, either. I wondered if it were possible that some of these men also had to use the men's room, but out of respect for proper etiquette, decided to wait it out. Was that why nobody moved a muscle? That seemed plausible. It also seemed like an impossible lead to follow.

My discomfort was building steadily. Again I looked back toward the exit.

Those three hundred eyes were still there, still focused on the podium like lasers. Of course, they weren't just any eyes. They belonged to the men who had collectively paid my tuition years earlier. But for their generosity, I wouldn't be in this room at all. Who knew how my life would have unfolded if Mr. Gerstell had told me to pack my bags and hit the road that day. These men not only played a critical role in my past, but they also now held the keys to the kingdom ... the keys to my future.

Now my past and future benefactors sat squarely between me and the men's room. Running this gauntlet in the middle of my boss's speech was certainly not the way to make a good impression. Had I really thought that winning them over was going to be a layup? Along with my cheesecake, I was now eating my words. If the gods were already punishing me for my gluttony, they might as well make me pay for my hubris, too.

Until somebody made a move, or until Si made his closing remarks, I was trapped. Panic set in as I struggled to batten down my backside. My imagination went into overdrive. What if I couldn't control my body? What if this former Scout remained in his seat, loyal and obedient—but not clean? Sadly I had a childhood memory of just such an occurrence.

When I was seven years old, I spent my first summer at Camp Hawthorne in Maine. I didn't make it to the toilet in time. Behind Cabin One, a wooded hill sloped down to Panther Pond, some sixty feet below. Vast and deep, the pond was the obvious place to discard my muddied briefs. No one would possibly find them there. After lights-out, I bravely went AWOL and snuck down to the water. I expected the pond's swift currents to whisk my tightey-not-so-whiteys away to distant shores like a message in a bottle. *Wouldn't it be hilarious if they washed up on the beach of our cross-pond rivals at Camp Timanous?*

The next morning, I heard bursts of laughter from behind the cabin. Walking down the hill, I asked what was so funny. The other campers had found a pair of soiled underwear floating in the water. *So much for reaching Camp Timanous.*

Confident that I couldn't be linked to the crime, I continued down the hill, where a small crowd had gathered.

"They're yours, aren't they?" Mark asked Brian.

"I didn't do it! I bet they're Bobby's," Brian said.

"Yeah, I think Bobby pooped his pants!" I joined in.

Seconds later silence fell over the mob. With a long stick, the underwear was lifted from the water for all to see. On the inside of the elastic band, printed in thick, black, indelible ink, the perpetrator was revealed: T. PHELAN. The laughter was as deafening as it was endless. I wanted to die.

Recalling this memory only heightened my inner tension. To those around me, I was sure I appeared no different from anybody else in the room: just another alumnus in a dark suit, white shirt, and red tie, politely listening to Headmaster Bunting tell us how well the Lawrenceville School was preparing its students to meet life's challenges.

Funny, I didn't recall being taught how to control my bodily functions during socially inopportune times. I suppose the closest we ever came to that was in a course called *Mind, Body, and Spirit*, when Mr. Smith tried to show us how to induce an out-of-body experience on command. Digging up that memory didn't help my current plight, either. Until I got to the men's room, the last thing in the world I wanted was to have an out-of-body experience.

The pressure from inside my body was overwhelming. Resisting such a powerful force seemed impossible. Like the finger in the dike, the strength of my sphincter was the only thing preventing a disaster. I continued to tighten my backside with all my might. I felt my heart pounding. A tingling sensation ran along the back of my upper thighs, and my thumbs and forefingers were slick with nervous perspiration. My breathing became shallow and rapid. I was terrified of humiliating myself—what if I couldn't successfully contain this juggernaut inside me? Yet at the same time, the thought of announcing my weakness by standing up and walking out was equally horrifying. *Damned if I do, damned if I don't.* I was screwed.

Eventually, after fifty-five agonizing minutes, my nightmare was close to over.

"Thank you very much." The ensuing thunderous applause served as confirmation. His speech had ended. I had been liberated. I was free. But I wasn't quite in the clear.

With tightly clenched butt cheeks, I stood up and began my precarious march across the cavernous room. I felt like a one-legged geriatric with a walker trying to hastily cross a busy six-lane freeway. My heart pounded. A bead of sweat trickled down my forehead.

Here it was, right in front of me, on a silver platter, as requested. The chance to mingle, to rub elbows, to make that great impression. But the introductions and the networking would have to wait—at least for the moment. I put my head down, avoided all eye contact, and plowed anonymously through the gauntlet.

By the time I returned, the crowd had dissipated. But thankfully all was not lost. A few stragglers remained. I checked my zipper, made sure my shirt was properly tucked in, and made a beeline in their direction.

Who were they? What exciting and lucrative lines of work were they in? I had to find out. This was my chance to salvage an otherwise disastrous day.

With a confident smile, I enthusiastically introduced myself to a pair of finely dressed, middle-aged men and listened in on the conversation already in progress.

"If crude oil prices keep skyrocketing, I'm going to have to rethink my strategy," one of the men lamented.

The other nodded. "My profits are completely dependent on what happens in the copper market."

I was riveted.

These guys must have been big-shot commodities traders down on Wall Street. Or maybe hedge fund managers, or senior executives at Exxon or Mobil.

I would soon learn that while in the men's room, I'd missed my golden opportunity. The high rollers were long gone. I spent the next half hour rubbing elbows with a gas station owner and, appropriately, a plumber. They were nice men and well educated, but I hadn't exactly hit the networking jackpot.

It was my second indication of the day that a Lawrenceville diploma was not a golden ticket to the good life.

At the time, I chalked the whole traumatic day up to a fluke, a mistake of my own making. I'd foolishly eaten too much, thrown caution to the wind by drinking coffee, and waited too long to answer nature's call. Under these circumstances, I thought, anybody would have found themselves in an equally dire situation.

I certainly didn't think anything was wrong with me. As with that humiliating Camp Hawthorne mishap so many years earlier, I figured, the memory of this day would eventually fade from my daily attention and be relegated to the harmless cellar of subconscious thought.

But in the meantime, it couldn't hurt to play it safe. After all, what was the Boy Scout motto? "Be prepared," right?

Three weeks later, we took Headmaster Bunting on the road again, hosting an identical event in Washington DC. This time around, I didn't have to worry about involuntary out-of-body experiences. I enjoyed every moment of his riveting speech—from my seat at the very back of the room, right next to the men's room.

They say that if a cat gets burned sitting on a hot stove, it will never sit on a hot stove again. But it will never sit on a cold one, either.

It wasn't an ideal adjustment, but I could live with that. As a bachelor who ordered a lot of pizzas, I didn't use the stove much anyway. I didn't realize at the time that there were many other ways to get burned in this world.

Hot Date

Nobody ever believed us. She was only three years older than I was, and we looked practically the same age. But as the youngest of my mother's four sisters, Missy was in fact my aunt. Born to have a career in sales, she worked in retail at the King of Prussia Mall outside Philadelphia. She was always looking out for me.

"Hey, it's your favorite aunt calling. Are you still single these days?" Subtlety was not her thing.

I had gone on a few dates here and there, but hadn't met anyone special to speak of. In the seven months I'd been living in New Jersey, my dating life had been painfully nonexistent—a sharp departure from my recent college days.

The sleepy town of Lawrenceville was far sleepier than I'd bargained for—hardly the ideal spot to meet young, single women. Nearby Princeton had plenty of female college students, but they socialized almost exclusively among themselves. I wasn't ready to get married, but having a steady girlfriend sure sounded appealing. To access any decent social scene, I basically had two choices: Philadelphia or New York.

"Yup, I'm still single, all right. Did you call to rub it in?"

"Hey, don't ever say I never did anything for you," she said. "I've got someone you need to meet. Her name is Kelly. She works with me. We're on for Saturday. It's all set up."

I never cared for blind dates, but there was a reason Missy had earned the title of my favorite aunt. She had a great track record in the matchmaking department and usually had a better idea of what I was looking for than I did. Thanks to Missy's introduction, I was already preapproved, just like the unsolicited credit card offers I'd recently started getting in the mail.

It took forty minutes to drive from my home to Pennsylvania, which meant that if things went well, this would be a commuting relationship. But after laying my eyes on Kelly, I didn't mind. I gladly would have driven a couple of hours to see a woman like her.

Kelly was twenty-two and five feet seven, with long, blond hair, and a pair of thighs so beautifully tanned and taut that the mere sight of them made me drool with desire. Not only was Kelly an absolute physical knockout, but she was also smart, independent, and wildly sarcastic. Without being high on herself, she exuded the confidence of a young woman who had it all together and knew that she was a great catch. *Thank you, Missy!*

During my college fraternity days, I had grown accustomed to having the upper hand with the women I dated. I typically called the shots. Being in Kelly's presence for only two minutes made me painfully aware that those days were gone. The post college world was different, and I was humbled to realize that I was once again a lowly freshman. Everything about how this woman carried herself suggested that she was no pushover. I would have to work to win her affection.

Pitched by Missy as a risk-free test drive, our first date was arranged as a double date. Missy's fiancé, Tom, would join us for an innocent, low-key afternoon in Valley Forge Park. No pressure, no obligation. We would have a picnic, throw the Frisbee around, and enjoy a beautiful spring afternoon under the sun. We took two cars. Kelly rode with Missy. Tom rode with me. If the date went well, then I would give Kelly a lift home.

The picnic was a success, and after two hours, I opened the car door for Kelly, and we were off. I must have done something right. Ah, another great first impression—with a little help from Missy. She had been the one who presold me to Kelly: *smart, funny, he's in great shape. Did I mention he's a triathlete? He's got a great job at this fancy boarding school. Trust me, he's a good guy.*

As we drove out of the park, I was excited that after just two hours, our meeting had morphed into a first date. Missy had no doubt hyped me up, but the fact that Kelly was now in my car suggested that I had at least come close to living up to that hype. Still, even though I had passed her initial screening criteria—whatever those were—I didn't feel as if I were securely in the driver's seat.

Kelly's striking good looks, combined with her confidence, were at once incredibly appealing and more than a little daunting. All I could think about was kissing her, and the still-immature, impatient frat boy in me didn't want to wait until our next date to do so.

Here was my dilemma: It was only four in the afternoon. Having your first kiss in broad daylight didn't seem right to me. Too awkward. Maybe grabbing an early dinner together would help extend this date into the evening. If I could buy just enough time to get past sunset, then I would greatly increase my odds of getting more than a handshake. Was I pushing my luck? Would she see right through my ploy? Would she think I was too aggressive? I didn't want to blow the deal, but I wanted to keep the momentum going. I couldn't help myself.

As I plotted my strategy, a low-grade disturbance developed in my gut. It was mild enough that, ordinarily, I might not have even given it a second thought. But since that disastrous alumni lunch in New York and a recent flight back from the West Coast, I was more tuned in to my digestive tract's babblings. At the slightest sign of gastric distress, I noticed, I was now much more vigilant about predicting when I would need to use a bathroom.

Given my new motto, "be prepared," this was an appropriate time to assess the seriousness of the rumblings by taking quick inventory of my bodily sensations. The threat did not appear to be in danger of escalating. *OK, nothing to worry about for now. False alarm.* My thoughts turned back to how I was going to get that kiss from Kelly.

"So, Missy said you do some traveling for work," Kelly said. "Have you been anywhere interesting yet?"

Uh-oh. Now what? More rumbling. A little spike in the pressure. Was it something I ate? Was it just me being nervous? Out of my peripheral vision, I could see a Sunoco gas station on our right. I was frozen with indecision. Should I play it safe? *Be prepared.* I ran another quick diagnostic check of my body. It was a tough call. I was not in a state of emergency, but inching in that direction.

"I just got back from San Francisco," I said.

The light turned green. I instinctively took my foot off the brake pedal and proceeded through the intersection. I turned my Volkswagen toward Route 202 North and accelerated onto the expressway, hoping I'd made the right decision. Once on 202, there was no going back. For better or worse, I was committed. Kelly's apartment was only ten minutes away. I was confident I could keep any out-of-body experience at bay for at least that long.

"Wow, how was that?"

"Are you kidding? I loved it," I said. "I'd never been out there before. It was so much fun that I ended up staying out there for the weekend. A couple of my high-school buddies live out there. We biked across the Golden Gate Bridge, ate lunch in Sausalito, and ran through the Presidio. It was amazing."

"I wish I could travel for business. It sounds so glamorous. I bet you just love it, don't you?"

I didn't want to tell her how I'd recently begun to feel about business travel. At a minimum, I'd sound like a whiner and a wimp.

Yes, I used to love it. I loved flying to Chicago and back. I even loved flying *to* San Francisco. As an avid fan of *Top Gun*, I turned every trip into my own private fighter-pilot fantasy, pretending the wide-body DC-10 was a sleek, supersonic F-14 Tomcat that I heroically maneuvered from my seat in coach.

But then I had that near miss on the return flight. I was trapped in seat 42-E like a compressed slice of white toast at the center of a club sandwich. Five ravaged dinner trays and four sleeping passengers held me in place like a toothpick, blocking the aisles to my right and left. I couldn't tell Kelly how the flight attendants' incessant chorus of

"Coffee? Coffee, ma'am? Sir, coffee?" dredged up a flashback of the New York luncheon with Si Bunting.

I hadn't even drunk any coffee, and I hadn't stuffed my face as I had in New York. I'd even made sure to use the men's room before getting on the plane. As far as I could tell, I hadn't done anything wrong. I *was* prepared!

It came out of the blue: the uncomfortably large carry-on bag—the kind with wheels—rolling rapidly down my digestive tract. Where did it come from? What would Kelly think if I told her that I'd almost used my seat cushion—not as a flotation device, as instructed in the safety demonstration, but as a toilet? Would she think less of me because I'd managed to avoid disaster only by "accidentally" spilling a cup of ice water on the poor guy dozing off in 42-F? Yes, I still dreamed of international travel and seeing the world, but that flight had left me adamantly unwilling to accept any seat assignment other than an aisle seat … or a toilet seat.

"Yeah, I do love it," I said, "but once you've done it a few times, it's not quite as glamorous as it's cracked up to be."

We were cruising down 202, going sixty-five or so, minutes from Kelly's apartment. Then, as was my habit, I started over thinking: *OK, Tim, even if you are able to hold it in until you reach Kelly's place, then what? Are you going to tell her you had a great time, then kick her out of your car so you can go find a public bathroom? What if she invites you up? "Hey, Kelly, great place! You don't mind if I lock myself in your bathroom, do you? Oh, by the way, do you have any matches?"*

I suppose bad smells eventually find reluctant acceptance in even the happiest long-term relationships. That said, they're a poor substitute for flowers, and no way to start a romance.

The more I thought about possible embarrassing outcomes, the more anxious I became. The more anxious I became, the more skittish my gut became. The forecast had dramatically changed; the threat level was climbing fast and there was a menacing storm on the horizon.

I gotta get off this freeway. Now.

We were approaching the junction of 202 North and I-76, the Schuylkill Expressway. Looking up the highway as far as I could, I saw traffic at a standstill. My car was exactly the place I didn't want to have an out-of-body experience. It would be one thing if I were alone in my car; it was quite another when I was driving with a beautiful woman whom I was trying to win over.

Doomsday scenarios raced through my mind. *What if we're stuck in traffic for a long time?* My feeling of urgency was growing. *What if I lose control of my body in my VW?* I would be humiliated, but Kelly would probably suffer more than me. Sitting in traffic, we wouldn't be moving fast enough to generate any fresh air blowing through the windows. We would be stuck in a hot, cramped, and malodorous Porta Potty. As far as all-time worst first dates go, this would have to be near the top of the list. *Hey, I had a great time today. Are you free next Friday? Let's take your car this time, OK?*

It didn't take me long to figure out what I had to do. If I wanted to have any shot at getting a second date with this woman, I needed to get off the highway before we hit the Schuylkill traffic. It wasn't going to be easy. The backup began less than a mile up the road, with only two exits ahead, and I was in the left lane doing about sixty-five. Nothing in the next lane resembled an opening.

It was as if my bowels had eyes of their own. They could see what we were up against. They knew the stakes were high. They were shouting at me and whipping me like a jockey coming down the stretch, doing everything they could to get this VW over to one of these two exits. *Come on, baby!* SMACK! *Come on, baby!* SMACK! *Gimme all you got!* SMACK! *You can do it!* SMACK!

Eliminating bodily waste is perfectly natural and necessary. However, unless you're living in a fraternity house, talking about it is not. Even I knew that no matter how euphemistically I might phrase it, this was not an appropriate topic for first-date conversation. Sharing with Kelly what I so urgently needed to do was incomprehensible. I was in mental and physical agony. Kelly was not only oblivious to my plight, but she was, in fact, trying to have a meaningful conversation with me.

"Don't they have a lot of earthquakes in San Francisco? Can you imagine anything more terrifying?"

"More terrifying than an earthquake?" I repeated.

Hmmm ... let me think about that one. How about the absolute fear of the humiliation I suspect I'm going to experience if I don't find a toilet in the next couple of minutes? Does that count?

"No. That would be horrible. I can't think of anything that would even come close."

This was a do-or-die situation. I squeezed into the right lane. Looking in the rearview mirror, I could read the driver's lips behind me. To accentuate his anger, he leaned on his horn. Then he flipped me off. His anger was well-founded, of course, but I was on a mission.

"Where are you going?" asked Kelly.

I was too preoccupied with getting off 202 to think about a plausible explanation for our sudden, unannounced freeway departure. *Where am I going? OK, time for some quick thinking. Come on, think of something. Anything but the truth.*

"Where am I going? Ahhh, I'm going to get off at this exit and take the back roads. I think it will be quicker with all the traffic up there."

Another quick snap of my head back and to the right. I turned my blinker on again. Another reckless—but successful—lane change. Another angry driver. Another middle finger.

Kelly wasn't buying it. "What's going on? Are you OK?" Was she angry or concerned? At this point, I didn't have time to figure it out.

I pulled into the exit lane and flew down the ramp. Not a gas station or a restaurant in sight. In front of us was an intersection. The stoplight had just turned red. Which way to safety?

OK, time to share a little more information.

"Am I OK? No, not really," I said. "I think I just drank too much water today, and I really have to go."

This wasn't a complete lie. I did have to go, but in my mind, there was a hierarchy to the business of bodily functions. Number one has always seemed more socially acceptable than number two. People don't usually seem disgusted by someone peeing on the side of the road, on the golf course, or behind a tree in a park.

But if polite society is somewhat tolerant of the public disposal of liquid waste, solids are an entirely different matter. Until you can find a restroom, you're pretty much expected to hold it in.

Of course, the rules are waived if you happen to be a dog. When nature calls our four-legged friends, they have the luxury of answering on the first ring. And nobody bats an eye. Their behavior is not only accepted—it's expected. As long as somebody has a pooper-scooper, the world is their toilet. How nice for them.

Kelly said I probably had chosen the worst exit to find a restroom. We sat at the red light for another minute. Now I was starting to panic. I tried to keep my composure. *Never let them see you sweat.* When the light turned green, I turned right. We found ourselves in front of some type of industrial warehouse facility.

"How about over there?" Kelly asked, pointing toward the building.

Since it was Saturday, maybe the place would be empty. I pulled into the parking lot. A row of shrubs and trees ran down the length of the building, acting as a divider from nearby railroad tracks. I threw the car into neutral and left the engine running. As I opened the door, I received a gift from the gods. A handful of paper napkins, left over from a recent trip to McDonald's, fell from the car onto the pavement. One less detail to worry about. Now things were starting to go my way. I grabbed the napkins off the blacktop, stuffed them into my pocket, and sprinted toward the shrubs.

Forty yards down my path, I ran into a snag. The shrubs and trees were not going to give me nearly enough privacy. Also, I was still in Kelly's direct line of sight. She'd know I wasn't peeing. She'd also know I had lied. I had to find a better spot and do it quickly. After all, guys don't take five minutes to pee in the bushes. She would get suspicious.

Directly across from my inadequate position among the shrubs was an empty loading dock that would be safely out of Kelly's sight.

Presumably the dock could also be used for *un*loading. No trucks. No workers. I dashed across the open space.

I walked back to the car with the trembling legs of a man who had just cheated death. *How in the world did I pull that off?*

"All better?" Kelly asked.

"Much better, thanks," I said, trying to sound nonchalant.

"Hey, I'm starting to get a little hungry. Feel like grabbing a drink and some dinner?" she asked.

"Sure, that sounds great."

A few hours later, with a kiss on the cheek and the promise of a second date, I drove off into the night. I had survived yet another rectal revolt physically unscathed—that was to say that I showed no outwardly visible signs of damage. Luckily Kelly never suspected a thing.

But this close call, like the others, left me rattled enough to make another adjustment to my normal behavior. After New York, I would only sit near the back of the meeting rooms. After my near miss at 35,000 feet in seat 42-E, I would avoid window and middle seats at all costs. After this date with Kelly, I became adamant about avoiding the traffic-choked highways that encircled her apartment in King of Prussia. If it could happen once, I figured, it could happen again. Maybe next time, I wouldn't be so lucky.

For our next few dates, I worked around this obstacle by inviting her to visit me in New Jersey. It was a convenient solution that lasted for about three weeks. But Missy and Tom's wedding presented an awkward scenario.

"I don't get it," Kelly said. "You're going to pass right by my apartment on your way to the church. Why can't you just pick me up?"

It was a legitimate question. It was a legitimate expectation. Our dating hadn't yet become serious, but that was no reason for me to shirk my duties as a gentleman. She wasn't asking for a lot—just the bare minimum, really.

I wanted to give her a ride. I wanted my family to see me walk into the church with her as my date. I really wanted to drive her home later that night. Still, I couldn't risk getting stuck again in that same traffic, on that same highway. I didn't know if I could trust my body.

Concocting some lame excuse about helping out with last-minute wedding details, I offered something along the lines of "Why don't I just meet you there?"

Kelly's response was terse. "Fine."

My efforts to cozy up to her before the ceremony, and later at the reception, couldn't have fallen flatter. I was in the doghouse. It was a disaster. In hindsight a simple explanation (albeit an embarrassing one) would have probably cleared everything up. It was conceivable that she might understand the traumatic impact of that abrupt pit stop. But no—at the time, such an admission would have been far too uncomfortable for me.

So, without any credible explanation from me, Kelly filled in the blanks, drawing her own conclusions. To a woman with plenty of eager suitors, my behavior was woefully unacceptable. I was a jerk who didn't care enough to treat her with the chivalry and respect that she deserved.

Nothing could have been further from the truth, but I couldn't bring myself to tell her that. I figured I was doomed no matter what I said.

In the end, I concluded that I'd prefer to have Kelly think of me as a complete ass rather than someone who's scared he can't control his ass. By my math, the charge of "failure to behave like a gentleman" carried slightly less shame and would allow me to hold on to a bit more of my dignity.

Only hours after Missy and Tom tied the knot, Kelly and I called it quits.

Connecting the Dots

I often used to wonder how I would feel when I heard the news. Given our past, I guess I didn't expect my reaction to be overly emotional. After the divorce, he and I were not close, seeing each other maybe once or twice a year during brief and sometimes uncomfortable holiday visits. The last time I'd seen my father was five months earlier in Colorado Springs, during Parents Weekend at the Air Force Academy, where my younger brother, Fred, was a freshman.

Before I got the news, I had planned on being in New Jersey with Lynn. It was Valentine's Day, 1990. We'd been dating for about three months, and I was looking forward to taking her out to dinner—somewhere even more romantic, perhaps, than TGI Friday's on Route 1.

But instead I was in Connecticut, in the small town of Darien. I'm not sure why, but I actually felt guilty asking for three days off from work. My boss, Andy, told me not to worry, assuring me this was more important; they would manage just fine without me for the next seventy-two hours.

My father had died of a heart attack. He was only fifty-one, but I was surprised that it hadn't happened sooner. I think everybody was. Even though I'd anticipated this moment, I was blindsided by the overwhelming flood of memories and feelings—both good and bad—that swirled through my head.

Part of me was angry that we were spending Valentine's Day—or any day, for that matter—at his funeral. This wasn't his first heart attack—more like his third or fourth, as I recall. The doctors had warned him time and again to stop smoking, eat better, lose weight, and start exercising. Why hadn't he listened?

But by the same token, I couldn't help but admire the spirit behind his devil-be-damned attitude. The guy suffered through multiple heart attacks, each time staring death squarely in the face as if playing a game of chicken with the Grim Reaper. Anybody in his right mind would do whatever he could to avoid going through that again. But that wasn't his style.

When it came to living, my father was a fierce advocate of quality over quantity. For better or worse, he was fearless. He didn't worry about consequences, much less about what people thought of him. He didn't spend much time pondering what-ifs. He had no interest in playing it safe—not in the stock market, not on the golf course, and not in the bar gambling with his backgammon buddies. If extending his life meant compromising his enjoyment of life, then he wanted no part of that trade. He didn't expect to live a long life, and that seemed to be just fine with him.

Our outlooks couldn't have been more different.

Not even the looming specter of death could get him to modify his behavior one iota. The fear of something far less ominous—the embarrassment of soiling myself—had caused me to make a handful of minor but noticeable changes to the way I lived my life. This would have been inconceivable to my father.

He would have scoffed at my adamant insistence on aisle seats. And my refusal to pick up Kelly simply because I might run into traffic and have an accident?

"What's wrong with you, son?" I can imagine him saying. "That's just crazy. Who cares what people think of you?"

Well, apparently I did. A lot. I wished I didn't. Life would be so much easier.

There were times when I would have given anything for my father's complete lack of self-consciousness, like on my second date with Lynn. After the Kelly fiasco, I endured a three-month dry spell before meeting someone I was really excited about.

Lynn had just graduated from college. She was living with her parents until she could find her own place. With the local dating pickings so slim, I couldn't afford to blow another great opportunity. I had to show her I was a gentleman.

When I picked her up at her parents' home, I was disappointed they were out for the evening. "Parent pleaser" was a role I played well, at least in the early stages of courtship.

While Lynn was upstairs blow-drying her hair, I searched for a place to tend to an untimely bout of indigestion—the direct result, I concluded, of the bottle of microbrewed beer that Lynn had graciously served me upon my arrival. Better to take care of my problem before we left for the movies, I figured. *Be prepared.*

I discovered a powder room off the foyer, right next to the front door. I opened the door and took a quick look around. It had everything I needed: a toilet, a full roll of toilet paper, running water, and, most important, a lock on the door. We were in business. The urgency was building to a crescendo.

It was at that precise moment, a split second before unleashing my sphincter, that I heard the voices. I froze. They came from outside. Whoever they were, they were coming closer. The voices grew louder as they approached the front door. Who could that be?

Two seconds later, I heard the sound of jiggling keys. The front door swung open.

"Hello? Lynn? Honey, are you still here? We're back, dear."

Wait. This wasn't right. Her parents were supposed to be out for the night. Lynn promised me they wouldn't be home until later. What happened? There I was, sitting on the john—*their* john—when they walked in. At least the powder-room door was locked. I decided to sit tight until they put their coats away and walked to another part of the house.

"Hi, Mom. Hi, Dad," I heard Lynn say. "Yeah, we're still here, but we're leaving for the movies in a minute."

"Where's your date?" whispered her mother, who had no idea that from my clandestine position, I was close enough to hear her heartbeat.

Thanks to the echo chamber created by the powder room's porcelain and tile, and the foyer's marble floor and high ceilings, I could hear her parents' every sound—and, I imagined, vice versa.

"Can we meet him and at least say hello before you head out?"

They'd heard good things about the young man who was taking their only child out for the evening. I did everything in my power to make sure they wouldn't hear ghastly things *from* him.

"Sure, but let me find him first," Lynn said. That was when she began to call my name out loud, as if looking for a runaway dog. "Tim? Tim? Where'd you go? Tim?"

I didn't want to give away my position by answering Lynn's calls. Everybody in the foyer would know my exact location soon enough—one way or another. It wasn't a question of if, but when. It was all academic at this point.

Meeting a woman's parents under normal circumstances was stressful enough. I was taking the game to a whole new level. This had turned into a standoff, and it was not going to end gracefully.

It was a curious time to have an entrepreneurial vision. If only the powder room had been built with soundproof technology, then I wouldn't be sweating this awkward situation.

That's it! It's genius! I will be the pioneer in creating the bathroom of the future. Yes, I will lead the masses to a bathroom from which no embarrassing noises can escape. The time-honored practice of running the water from the faucet to drown out embarrassing noises will be a thing of the past. I won't just build new noise-absorbing bathrooms, but people will line up to have me retrofit their existing bathrooms, too. I'm going to be rich! Of course, I will need to put together a business plan and line up some investors ...

My daydream came to an abrupt end when I briefly and suddenly lost control of my sphincter. My body was hell-bent on performing for the unsuspecting audience.

A short blast echoed throughout the powder room, followed in rapid succession by several more. With acoustics that rivaled those of the Hollywood Bowl, each note, both high and low, ricocheted off the porcelain and reverberated through the adjacent amphitheater. I felt my face turn bright red. My eyes lit up like headlights.

It was out there. Oh God.

I remembered a phrase from my high-school French class. *Les jeux sont faits.* Roughly translated, it means *the game is up.*

My body tensed up as I waited for my audience's reaction. The conversation came to a brief halt. *Uh-oh.* For several seconds, I heard only silence. Then the talking resumed.

I breathed a sigh of relief. Immediately following that sigh was a deafening follow-up of epic proportions. It wasn't just loud. This burst had hang time. Not even counting the ensuing echo, the blast continued uninterrupted for four … full … long … seconds.

No way would that one go unnoticed. The echoes continued to ricochet throughout the amphitheater. I was so embarrassed that I began quietly to laugh.

Big mistake.

My chuckle took away any semblance of control I had left over my body. I wish I could have seen the looks of horror on the three faces on the other side of the door. The second explosion dwarfed the first in both volume and duration—to say nothing of the smell. It reeked so badly that it was making *me* cringe, which is rare.

Everyone could hear the performance clearly. Pavarotti was playing the Bowl, and the tenor was just warming up. *Stick around, folks. You ain't heard nothin' yet. If you liked that, you'll love this.*

Ten minutes later, the concert came to a close. The tenor had nothing left to give the audience. There would be no encores tonight. The Bowl grew silent. I was drained.

After a thorough hand washing, the time had come. I couldn't procrastinate anymore. If the powder room had had a window, I would have crawled out and driven off into the night. Digging a tunnel, à la *The Great Escape*, would take too long. The only way out of this room was through the door.

I looked in the mirror. Just as I thought, my face was bright red with embarrassment. How was I going to look her parents in the eye?

How was I going to shake hands with them? Would they be offended if I tried? Unfortunately the reluctant tenor would have to step outside and face the music. It was time to please the parents.

I walked out to an empty hall. Lynn and her parents were gathered in the kitchen.

"Hi, you must be Tim. I'm Steve Waverly," said Lynn's father, as he stood up and extended his hand. "It's nice to meet you."

"We've *heard* ..." her father continued, with a pause that was too long to be unintentional, "a lot about you."

I was horrified. What could I possibly say?

"Only good things, I hope," I replied.

An embarrassing moment, to be sure. Happily the rest of the date went just fine, as did the next one, and the one after that.

The only lessons I drew from that face-reddening mini drama were the obvious ones: The rich flavor of microbrewed beer didn't agree with me. *So, dummy, don't drink microbrewed beers.* Common sense. This was just one more isolated incident that, by unfortunate coincidence, happened to involve an untimely protest from my digestive tract.

Not that I was counting, but my first date with Lynn marked my fourth untimely bodily crisis. Two had occurred at work, the other two on dates. Only one involved coffee, cheesecake, and overeating. Only one involved a microbrew. Yes, before each of the dates, I had been a little nervous. But on the plane and at the alumni luncheon, I hadn't been nervous or panicky until after my bowels started acting up.

Aside from the fact that all four episodes had come within a fairly short period of time—I'd only been out of college for about a year and a half—I wasn't aware of any common denominator that linked these close calls together. It never even occurred to me to look for one. These had been nothing more than four random cases of bad luck. End of story.

But if that was all there was to it, then why was I having these thoughts at my father's viewing, the night before his funeral?

I needed to know all the details about the next day, every last one. My mom didn't pick up on it. She probably thought it was more of the same; from the time I could first talk, I had an annoying habit of demanding specific and precise responses to my questions.

My mother, by contrast, was seemingly allergic to detail, always attempting to dismiss my inquiries with explanations that were blatantly fabricated and utterly devoid of any pertinent specifics. But my questions were not more of the same. Far from it.

I knew that we would all meet at the funeral home the next morning and drive to the church. My mother said the church was in Stamford, the next town over.

"Yes, I realize that, but where exactly?"

"I don't know, Tim. I've never been there before."

"How long will the drive take? Do we have to follow the hearse?"

"Probably ten or fifteen minutes, maybe. I'm really not sure."

She was losing patience, so I backed off. I still had so many questions that needed to be answered. Would we be driving to the church on the back roads or on I-95? How long would the church service last? Which route would we take to the cemetery? How long would we be there?

I didn't tell anybody, but I was now obsessed with knowing in advance the likelihood of locating a toilet at a moment's notice. Sure, after each previous episode, I'd taken steps to ensure that I wouldn't repeat my mistakes. But now I was looking into the future, trying to anticipate new threats that hadn't even materialized yet. This was definitely a new and unwelcome wrinkle.

I was surrounded by friends and family. It wasn't like I was concerned about impressing them. The only person who I would have liked to impress was the man lying peacefully in the open casket at the front of the room. What did he really think of me? Now that he was gone, I found myself revisiting another complicated question: what did I think of him?

Over the years, it had been the painful memories and his shortcomings that automatically popped into my head when I thought of my father. When things were bad, they were really bad—and often the direct result of his inability to control his alcoholism.

My default memories were of late-night police visits, missed birthdays, and the sudden financial insolvency that forced my newly single mother to raise three children with no assistance—monetary or otherwise. The screaming and fighting between them hadn't happened all the time, of course—only when he came home. Even when I was in third grade, I had a pretty good idea that this wasn't what marriage was supposed to be like.

In those two days before the funeral, everybody had an amusing anecdote or two to tell about my father. I guess I had forgotten that when he wasn't drinking, people loved being around him, probably because he embraced life so aggressively.

For years, he had been a good provider—a great provider, as a matter of fact. When he met my mom, she was a young, divorced mother of two. He married her and legally adopted my younger sister, Lisa, and me, choosing to raise us as his own. From the time I was two, I called him Dad. When Fred was born a year later, we seamlessly became the Phelan family.

All's right in my world whenever I can put everything into a neat little box or category. Gray areas and loose ends drive me crazy. The hours we spent in the funeral home reminded me that defining a person can be tricky business; judging somebody can be much harder still.

My dad was weak, strong, and flawed. He started heroically but finished less than admirably. Even if my father didn't realize or acknowledge it, actions have consequences. Living for the moment, as if there's no tomorrow, comes with consequences. From my vantage point, his carefree attitude was partly responsible for our turbulent childhood, the riches-to-rags story, and the failure of a once-promising marriage. Those weren't accidents. They were consequences.

In almost every sense, the way I lived my life was a perfect opposite reaction to how my father had lived his. More than resentment, the memories from my roller-coaster childhood motivated me to do things differently.

Like him, I would build my own financial fortune. But I would make sure to protect it, so that when the proverbial rainy day came along, I would be prepared.

I definitely wanted to get married, but only once. I would take my time, do my homework, and shop around for my perfect wife. My marriage would be divorce-proof. My family would enjoy a comfortable lifestyle, but not lavish. My children would be well taken care of, but not spoiled. They would have all of life's necessities, but few, if any, of its excesses.

All I wanted was stability, comfort, and happiness. And by the time I graduated from college, it was all within reach. I didn't know exactly how it was going to unfold, but I was confident that everything would fall into place.

And if there was one thing I was sure of, it was that I wasn't going to let myself die young—especially from a heart attack.

After losing forty-five pounds during my junior year in college (my primary motivation at the time was to be noticed by more women), I entered my first triathlon on a whim. One race quickly led to another, and before long I was spending huge chunks of each day swimming, biking, and running. I thrived on the competition, secretly wondering if this once-fat couch potato might someday become a professional triathlete. If nothing else, being fit would increase my odds of meeting women and decrease my odds of dying prematurely.

◆　　　◆　　　◆

The drive from the funeral home to the church was tense. I had been told that the family—eight or nine of us, anyway—would ride in a stretch limousine. Inside the car, there were tears, and choking to hold back the tears. My throat was constricted, and my insides were in knots. I looked out the window, scoping out the residential streets of Stamford. *Who lives in these houses? Are they the kind of people who might allow a nicely dressed, grieving stranger into their home for a brief pit stop?*

When we arrived at the church, I immediately bolted for the men's room. Because I was one of the pallbearers, my trip needed to be a quick one. I had responsibilities. People were counting on me.

Outside the church, the funeral director reminded us to carry the coffin, which was the heaviest object I had ever lifted in my life, carefully and slowly into the church and up to the altar.

After a traditional hour-long Catholic Mass, the other pallbearers and I reconvened to escort the coffin back to the hearse—again, carefully and slowly. The second that was done, I ran back inside to use the toilet again. Again I didn't have much time. The procession was ready to leave. I sprinted back into the limo, where my family had been wondering where I was and why I was taking so long.

We reversed our original path through the same suburban streets, so I didn't have to waste any mental energy wondering if there might be any public facilities along the way. I now knew there were not. Nonetheless the ride was quicker than I expected. Before I knew it, we passed through the cemetery's tall iron gates.

When I stepped outside, it was damp, gray, and dreary. If it were a few degrees colder, it would have been snowing instead of drizzling.

The last cars in the procession pulled up and turned off their motors. The graveside service was about to get under way. This would be it—my last chance to pay my respects. My last chance to say good-bye. Regardless of our past, the last thing I wanted to do was tarnish this ceremony in any way. This was not a moment I wanted to miss; I would never be able to forgive myself.

But my bowels didn't want to cooperate. They were kicking and screaming. My head swiveling, I made a desperate survey of the cemetery grounds. There were plenty of trees, but I didn't want to be involved in any act of desecration. I didn't feel like going to jail ... or, for that matter, to hell.

Everybody was gathered around the plot, and the only sounds were of sniffling. I walked over and stood next to my brother, my sister, and my mom. My brother reached out to hold my hand. I grabbed it and squeezed tightly. The priest began his prayer.

I was a mess. I knew that I should be consumed with grief. But I couldn't help it: my father was not the only thing on my mind. While the priest made some heartfelt comments and gave his blessing, I stared off into the distance.

Three or four hundred yards in front of me, on the busy Post Road, I saw a gas station. Even from this distance, I could make out the Men and Ladies signs on the doors. I should have been a pilot—my eyes were great. *How long would it take me to run over there?*

The soldiers in military honor guard fired their rifles three times. The ceremony was almost over. Still I couldn't stop staring at the gas station. I felt so guilty.

The bugler played "Taps," and everyone started to cry, including me. Despite my best efforts, I was still having trouble focusing on mourning. I didn't want to say good-bye, but I couldn't wait for the ceremony to be over. How inappropriate.

What's wrong with me? Why is my body doing this to me?

I entertained the theory that maybe this was the work of my subconscious. Had it put these previously unconnected close calls together like pieces of a jigsaw puzzle, looking for a pattern, an answer? That didn't make sense; I thought my subconscious was designed to keep me safe and out of danger.

Frankly, I didn't know what to think anymore. I couldn't find any easy answers, and I couldn't put this into a box.

I couldn't stop thinking about it. When would it happen again? And where would I be when it happened? Traffic and middle seats were one thing, but I couldn't very well avoid family funerals in the future, could I?

Four Square Miles
Surrounded by Reality

I gasped for air. It felt as if a grenade were about to explode through my chest. My muscles were screaming, burning from fatigue—especially my arms. I needed to rest. Fifteen seconds was not enough. My teeth chattered uncontrollably. It was probably sixty degrees, but it felt more like forty.

The second hand swept up toward the top of the pace clock. Only three more seconds. Another quick mouthful of oxygen. Then we were off. The shivering stopped. The water in the pool was much warmer than the air.

For the next two and a half minutes, I propelled myself up and down the twenty-five-yard lane eight more times, struggling to keep pace with the six swimmers in front of me. We would spend the next hour and a half repeating this sprint-then-rest routine. It hurt like hell, but I told myself that this would take me to the next level; this was why I was there.

As if to remind me of what was next on my to-do list, the early morning sun shone brilliantly on the Flatirons, Boulder's signature trio of vertical, sheer faced rock formations on the west side of town. They looked like giant arrowheads pointing to the sky. Just behind these jagged rocks, the foothills of the Rockies rose abruptly toward the 14,000-foot, snowcapped peaks in the distance.

After swim practice and a bite to eat, I would join some friends for a five-hour, eighty-mile bike ride into the mountains' steep, twisting canyons. If I timed it right, I would still be able to squeeze in a quick five-mile run before sunset.

To those who compete in these swim-bike-run races, triathlons are grueling tests of speed, strength, endurance, and mental toughness. To the rest of the world, this relatively obscure sport probably looks more like a senseless exercise in masochism. Count my mom as a member of the latter group. I remember when I first told her about my new career path.

"What about those nice offers you got from those Lawrenceville people?" she asked. "I don't know about that manufacturing job, but you can make a very comfortable living working for that big insurance company. The import-export thing also sounded exciting. Are you sure you don't want to call them back?"

She was right. I had passed up some offers that would have put me on the fast track to suburban-home ownership and country-club living. What was I thinking? My mom was scared that I might be derailing my professional plans.

"Don't you still want to go into international business?" she asked.

"Mom, look, I'm still going to do all that. Don't worry. This is just something I need to get out of my system. It's only for a year or two."

"But why can't you do the triathlon thing *and* still have a good job?" she persisted. "How are you going to eat and pay rent?"

She had always been a worrier, but in this case, I understood her concern. After the divorce, with three kids and no child support, she had gone to heroic lengths—she worked two jobs while going back to school to earn her college degree—to make sure we turned out OK.

She had learned how to dig down and make tough sacrifices so we could get by. And for what? So her oldest son could follow a pipe dream of becoming a professional athlete in a sport where only a dozen people make a comfortable living? Clearly this wasn't the future she had envisioned for me. But, as always, she remained supportive.

"I can't do this halfway," I said. "I need to train full time. I'll wait tables at night if I have to. Like I said, it's not going to be forever."

I told myself I was merely putting one dream on hold while I pursued another one that was more time-sensitive. I was in my athletic prime, free of the time constraints and financial obligations that came with being a responsible adult. In a few years, I would have a stable career, a wife, two or three kids, and a mortgage.

But at the time, I had potential. And I didn't want to look back years later and wonder if I could have made it.

"Besides, I'll be close to Fred," I'd explained.

Boulder was less than two hours away from Colorado Springs, where my younger brother was about to start his second year at the Air Force Academy. I figured we could both use some family nearby, especially now that Dad was gone.

My mom couldn't argue with that. She and my stepfather, John—they'd been happily married for about seven years—had recently moved to London for John's job. They'd be there for two years.

◆   ◆   ◆

Swimming, biking, and running. Eating and sleeping.

Each day I rose before the sun, a tough competitor who thrived on pushing himself to the outer edges of his physical and mental limits, bravely exploring the human thresholds of pain and fatigue in a relentless quest to wring every last ounce of extractable performance from his being.

Impressive, isn't it?

Most people seemed to think so.

Of course, I was aware of the contradiction. I knew all too well what nobody else would ever suspect: over the last few years, I hadn't exactly been the poster boy for living a courageous life.

Everything I told my mother about why I wanted to pursue a triathlon career was true. This was something I was passionate about. But I didn't tell her that by chasing my dream, I was also running from my fears. At the time, I don't know if I admitted that to myself.

After my father's funeral, I looked at the world in a whole new way.

Every day I was sure that another ambush was always around the next corner. I felt like a moving target, living my life in between the crosshairs of a trigger-happy sniper who watched my every move, day and night, just waiting for the chance to attack my dignity and take me down when I least expected it.

Being prepared wasn't enough. I had to live in the future, often days or weeks down the road. The key to survival was anticipating and avoiding all threats *before* they materialized. Unfortunately taking such precautions came with its own consequences.

In my final months working at Lawrenceville, I was back in Manhattan and running late for a meeting. Catching the express subway, something I'd routinely done hundreds of times, was my only chance.

Instead I opted for the slower local train. Stopping every twenty or thirty seconds, the local gave me better odds of jumping off to find a bathroom en route. When I arrived a half hour late for the meeting, the receptionist shook her head and suggested I reschedule.

What were my chances of becoming an international business tycoon if I couldn't master a mundane, twelve-minute ride on the New York subway?

A month later, I was still in New Jersey, pondering my career options, when I opened the envelope from my mom. It was a stack of snapshots and a short note.

Dear Tim,

London is fantastic! I took these around our new neighborhood. You'll love all the history, the architecture, and the culture (the food could be better). I can't wait to show you everything. Maybe you can come over this summer?

Love, Mom

I wasn't necessarily dying to see England, but France was practically next door. I could perfect my French with the help of the Parisian women (I was newly single after Lynn moved to Boston a month earlier).

She probably shouldn't have sent me the pictures. London's narrow streets and buildings looked historic, all right. Actually, ancient would be a better description. The photos suggested a city with nothing in the way of public, modern restrooms. I didn't see a single convenience store, not one gas station.

But an even bigger hurdle was the journey itself.

I wasn't crazy about the idea of a seven-hour overseas flight and what I expected to be an inadequate passenger to lavatory ratio in coach. I could just picture the horrifically long lines. I'd be a sitting duck. And with my luck, this would all go down in the first hour, leaving me to endure another four or five hours in my soiled state before landing. And what about customs? "Anything to declare, sir?" God, they'd probably bring the dogs in to sniff around.

I had no illusions that these were rational thoughts. The whole thing was nuts, and I suspected I was some kind of a head case. I was pretty sure everybody else would, too. Knowing my mom, she'd chalk my fears up to poor mothering. She didn't need anything else to worry about. How could I begin to explain something so silly and, at the same time, so scary?

"Sorry, Mom. Work is going to be crazy until the middle of July, and then I'm racing until September. Maybe I could come in October? November, maybe?"

I'm not sure what made me feel worse—passing up this opportunity, or lying to my mother about why I was passing it up. I could have found time to get away. And I also could have found time to pursue my triathlon dream while holding down a full-time job. It wasn't about the time.

It was about business meetings, luncheons, planes, and express subway rides. All the good jobs (all the ones I knew about, anyway) required these kinds of things. And, for the moment anyway, I'd lost the confidence to handle these mundane background tasks.

Packing up my VW and moving to Boulder seemed like my best option. I'd be back ... right after this freak storm passed by. I just needed a time-out.

◆   ◆   ◆

Boulder has a well-deserved reputation as a haven for Birkenstock-wearing, tree-hugging, free spirits who embrace all things liberal, holistic, and antiestablishment.

The town is often described as four square miles surrounded by reality. For a traditional, clean-cut kid from the New York suburbs, it was an unlikely place to find tranquility.

I spent my nights working at the Walnut Brewery. As a waiter, I was never trapped in any situation for longer than the two or three minutes it took to rattle off the dinner specials and explain to one dismayed tourist after another that our *brew pub* brewed its own beer and, regrettably, did not serve Budweiser.

Similarly, during swim practice, the locker room was never more than thirty yards away. Most of my running and cycling training was in the heavily wooded, sparsely populated foothills of the Rockies—a sprawling, open-air men's room that never had a line.

Besides being a magnet for aging hippies, hippie wannabes, and college kids, Boulder was also the mecca for triathlon training. Every day I got the chance to train alongside the sport's elite—my idols. Shortly after moving to town, I found myself sharing the swim lane with a living legend.

In its 1982 broadcast of the famed Hawaii Ironman competition, ABC Sports captured what remains arguably the sport's most defining moment. Julie Moss, having already swum 2.4 miles, biked 112, and run all but the final hundred yards of the 26.2-mile marathon, succumbed to exhaustion and dehydration. After scraping herself off the pavement, Julie staggered heroically toward the finish line while keeping only sporadic control over her fatigued legs—and her bowels. The cameras caught every moment of her dramatic, courageous, and colorful second-place finish and televised it for the world to see—freshly darkened running shorts and all.

To this day Julie Moss, feces-stained runner-up, enjoys unwavering idol status throughout the triathlon world. What other career would tolerate, let alone applaud, a self-soiling second-place finish? I had every reason to believe that I could reach the top in this sport.

If Boulder didn't completely insulate me from reality, it sure came close. As I had hoped, my bowels took an instant liking to their new surroundings. In fact, they'd never been happier.

Since leaving New Jersey, I didn't miss my old reality a bit. Virtually every day I spent in the cozy little cocoon of Boulder was a day without digestive problems. I decided that I never wanted to leave. This would be my home.

But to avoid going back to the real world, I had to do two things: go fast enough to make a living as a pro, and find a woman who would be willing to spend the majority of her remaining years inside Boulder's city limits.

◆　　◆　　◆

My training ride up to Rocky Mountain National Park and back took almost six hours. I was running on empty, my calves and quadriceps throbbing and sapped. Exhausted, famished, and parched, I relied on gravity to guide me the last two miles to my apartment.

I don't know how I even saw her in the first place. I was coasting speedily down the Broadway hill toward the Pearl Street mall; she was riding her bike up the path in the opposite direction, toward the CU campus. But in that blur, I just knew it was her—the cute waitress from the Mexican restaurant. *What was her name? Sarah? I think that's what she told me. Yes, I'm sure that's it. Sarah.*

If I had stopped to think about it, I doubt I would have traversed four lanes of briskly moving traffic to pursue a girl who, in all likelihood, wouldn't even remember me. But when I saw that blonde ponytail bobbing up and down, I didn't have a choice. This was one of those adrenaline-driven, primal reactions where instinct took over, trumping all logic and reason.

In the blink of an eye, I was weaving through the oncoming traffic, dodging the crisscrossing steel and rubber like a crazed, kamikaze Manhattan bike messenger.

Where'd she go?

As I sprinted up the bike path, I saw her golden ponytail cresting the hill. I was gaining on her.

Faster, faster.

With her petite, slender frame and taut, athletic calves, she looked fit. *Probably a runner*, I thought. But my eyes were drawn back to her bouncing hair, now only twenty yards in front of me.

Like a dog that suddenly runs down the car he never really expected to catch in the first place, I wasn't exactly sure what to do next. *You caught her. Now slow down. You don't want to look desperate. Catch your breath, and think of something intelligent to say.*

When she stopped at the crosswalk, I pulled alongside her. We waited for the light to change, just the two of us. *Come on, think of something to say. Anything.*

"Hey, you work at Rio, don't you?" I asked. It wasn't my best stuff, but I wanted her to think this was a chance encounter, not the spontaneous stalking it actually was. "I think you waited on me the other night."

"Wait a minute … were you with that big group of girls?"

"Good memory." I wanted her to know I was single. "That was my sister and her friends. By the way, my name's Tim."

She smiled and reached for my hand. "I'm Sarah."

I knew it!

Two nights later, I went back to Rio and asked Sarah out. Within a week, we became inseparable. Within a year, we were sharing a bedroom—and a bathroom, too.

◆   ◆   ◆

My season had gotten off to a solid early start. In Phoenix, Vermont, and Tampa, I had turned in a series of top-ten amateur finishes. And as the season moved into the summer, my hard work was paying off. I narrowed the gap even more between me and the pros. I was on a roll.

Back on the home front, nine months of unwedded cohabitation had given Sarah and me a pretty good glimpse into the joys, as well as the challenges, of married life. For the most part, we got along great, and living with Sarah was as easy as it was enjoyable.

"She's a very sweet girl, Tim," my mother said to me after visiting us. "Do you think you'll end up marrying her?"

"I don't know, Mom. We don't really talk about it."

"You've been dating for, what, almost two years?" she said. "You better start talking about it. She's not going to stick around forever. What are you waiting for?"

"Mom, calm down," I said. "Talking about marriage is a little premature at this point. Remember, Sarah still has another semester of college left. Who knows what she's going to want to do after graduation?"

"And what about you?" she asked. "How much longer are you going to do this triathlon thing?"

"Well, it all depends on how I do in Cleveland," I told her. "If I finish in the top twelve, then I'm going to turn pro and stay here in Boulder."

"And if you *don't* make the top twelve?"

"Honestly, that's not an outcome I really want to think about," I said. "But I guess I'd call it quits and figure out my next career move."

"John and I will be back from London in a few months. Do you think you'd consider moving back East?"

"I don't know, Mom. Let's just see how the race goes, all right?"

◆   ◆   ◆

I called Sarah the night before the race.

"How do you feel? Excited?" she asked.

"I am excited. But nervous, too," I said. "I've never seen a field this strong. Seriously, *everybody's* here for this race. I've got my work cut out for me, that's for sure."

Cleveland was that year's site for the National Amateur Championships. The top twelve finishers in each age group would earn the chance to represent the United States at the World Triathlon Championship in Sydney, Australia. Obviously, even if I did make the team, I wasn't sure I could bring myself to make *that* flight. For me, qualifying for the team offered a greater reward: the green light to turn pro.

"You've been racing well all year," Sarah said, "and I think you have a great chance of pulling it off."

"Thanks. I hope you're right," I said. "Anyway, enough about me. Any news on your end?"

With graduation only a few months away, Sarah had been doing a lot of on-campus job interviews—"just to keep all my options open," as she explained it. I was hoping she would want to stay in Boulder, and she knew it.

"I got asked back for a second interview with that accounting firm in Chicago," she said. "Don't worry ... I'm probably not going to get it. And even if they do make me an offer, I have no idea if I'll take it."

"Well, congratulations on getting to the next round. That's exciting," I said, trying to sound more enthusiastic than I had when she'd told me about the first interview. "I better get off the phone and try to get some sleep. I'm going to need it."

It was unsettling to realize how much of my fate was out of my hands. I couldn't make Sarah stay in Boulder. Nor did I have any say over how fast my competitors would race. The only thing I had any control over was the performance of my own body ... but even that was iffy.

◆   ◆   ◆

The alarm clock went off at four. I was disoriented. *Where am I?* Then I remembered. Cleveland. *But why?* Oh yeah, the race. But that was the fun part. That was later.

It was what I had to deal with beforehand that was going to suck. It always did.

Even though daybreak was still an hour away, my bowels, like any self-respecting workaholics, were up and rarin' to go. Jet lag? Insomnia? Those terms meant nothing to them. After all, they knew it was race day. Things were always different on race day.

Only minutes after my first urgent trip to the bathroom, my body demanded a second. By any measure, the workaholics had turned out a full week's work. It was mind-boggling to realize they were just getting warmed up.

Apparently my digestive tract operated by the same physics-defying phenomenon that allowed me to continue extracting toothpaste from the tube for weeks after I had declared it empty. It was never *truly* empty, not in any definitive way. It made no sense.

Part of the explanation had to be nerves and the gallons of adrenaline pouring through my veins. But nerves alone couldn't explain a week's worth of output in just over ten minutes. I figured the ungodly amount of food I ate each day to fuel my training must also play a role. The more I put into my body, the more would come out.

As I made my predawn drive through the Cleveland suburbs, the familiar tingling sensations inching north of my upper hamstrings told me that my little workaholics were in no mood to take a break. And, as usual, time was of the essence.

I passed lots of service stations and restaurants, but they were all closed. On the off chance that I might stumble across a restroom up ahead, I decided to keep driving for a mile or so.

The workers were getting antsy. I could feel the complex machinery of my gastrointestinal tract begin to churn. Seconds later, the factory bristled with activity. After the morning's production, where would they possibly get the raw materials to manufacture even one speck more? Surely even this factory had a daily limit, no? Miraculously they were able to produce this stuff seemingly out of thin air.

It was like going to the circus and wondering how so many clowns could possibly pop out of that one tiny car ... but trust me, it wasn't nearly as entertaining.

As I did on the way to most races, I was going to have to ditch. It was an unpleasant part of my prerace routine, but at least it was predictable.

I pulled over next to an open field. It was quiet and dark. I strategically positioned myself between my rental car and the fence, so I could spare any approaching motorists the horror of beginning their morning with the sight of my unseemly transgression.

I also prayed the police wouldn't drive by. If I had to guess, I was violating at least a couple of laws. For starters, littering and indecent exposure came to mind. Surely a good attorney could make a compelling case that I was forced to do this, against my will—like Patty Hearst.

As I peeled away from the scene of the crime, my headlights illuminated one of those Adopt a Highway signs: "This mile sponsored by Girl Scout Troop 213." I made a mental note: *Buy many, many boxes of their cookies.*

By six o'clock, I got to the start area, where the race organizers had once again failed to grasp the basic concept of supply and demand. It didn't take an economics major to figure out what would happen when you combined two thousand triathletes with only ten portable toilets.

By six forty-five, the start area buzzed with activity. Tension and nervous energy permeated the humid morning air. Most triathletes had Type A personalities. Bikes were tuned, tires pumped, water bottles filled, and muscles stretched.

A quick glance at my Timex. Seven o'clock. As I laid out my gear, the tri-geek next to me boasted about his latest equipment purchase. Triathletes loved to talk about their high-tech, lightweight gadgets.

"See these titanium wheel hubs? They make my bike three hundred grams lighter."

Three hundred grams lighter? If I had more time, I would tell him how, that morning, I had already lost two or three *pounds*—and I wasn't done yet.

From my backpack I retrieved my strategically stashed toilet paper and headed for the woods. As with all my other toilet trips that morning, this one would not be in vain. Nor would it be my last.

By the time I stepped up to the starting line, I had made four *more* trips to the woods. In three and a half hours, I had relieved myself eight times. Eight!

◆   ◆   ◆

With an ear-piercing horn blast, the race of my life began.

Three seconds later, the lightly rippling waters of Lake Erie turned frothy and violent as more than a thousand swimmers jockeyed for position, thrashing their way toward the first buoy, some seven hundred yards away. From above, the scene resembled a ferocious feeding frenzy of Great Whites. From my perspective, it looked no different.

Swallowing a few mouthfuls of nasty lake water was unavoidable. So were the kicks to my head and someone's occasional attempt to swim directly over me. The morning sun reflected off the water and right into our eyes. It was impossible to spot the first buoy. I put my head down and kept sprinting.

As always happened by this point in a race, my gut and my backside were finally silent. But I knew they weren't empty—just distracted. If history was any guide, they would stay that way for at least another two hours.

Out of the water and onto the bike, I managed to catch the leaders by mile ten. That was when I *really* put the hammer down. I only had fifteen miles to put as much time on the field as I could before I started the run. Some of these guys were great runners. We're talking thirty-three minutes for 6.2 miles—that was like 5:20 per mile. Lightning.

Running was my weakest event. On a great day, I *might* be able to hold 5:50 per mile. Maybe. But by mile four, I was having an awesome run. By my standards, I was positively hauling ass. I wasn't in the lead, but right in the mix. Only two miles left.

Rounding the back of Municipal Stadium, I kicked it into high gear. Less than a quarter mile to go.

As I dug down deeper, my heart rate spiked to its redline. One hundred yards left.

I sprinted across the finish line and looked up at the clock. One hour and fifty-four minutes. A career personal best—I had never gone faster. It was an exhilarating feeling and one hell of a performance.

Grabbing a cup of Gatorade, I walked over to check out the official results. It didn't take me long to spot my name, time, and finishing place posted on the fifteen-foot-high bulletin board.

As waves and waves of my competitors rolled toward the finish, I made my way over to a pay phone. I had news to deliver.

Makin' Copies

On the other end of the phone, my mom struggled to suppress her glee. She was relieved to learn that her twenty-seven-year-old, college-educated son was now free to get what she referred to as a real job. After four years of earning $18,000 per year waiting tables at the Walnut Brewery, I was excited about the possibility of once again earning a real *salary*.

As I would quickly discover, this was easier said than done. Boulder was a town where PhDs were willing to work as Safeway checkout cashiers in exchange for the privilege of living in this picturesque town at the foot of the Rockies. Searching the help-wanted ads yielded nothing. I was actually laughed out of employment agencies for trying to find a job that paid more than $25,000 per year. I was beginning to think I would never catch my big break.

Jeff was a regular customer at the brewery. He usually sat in my section, and we had a good rapport. He was five years older than I was and always came in wearing a suit and tie. Since our lunchtime conversations typically revolved around discussing politics and trading sophomoric jokes, I never got around to asking him what he did for a living. Given my bleak prospects, I posed the question.

"Funny you should ask," he said. As it turned out, he owned a company that sold office copiers to local businesses. A natural-born salesman, Jeff knew precisely what bait to put on the hook. "I just started looking for a new salesman, and I think this job is something you'd be great at." He was selling me, and I didn't even realize it. "Interested in working for me?"

How could I not be? With mounting debt and a depleted savings account, I was eager to get my professional life back on track. And let's face it: "I used to be a triathlete, but now I just wait tables" wasn't going to get me too far with the ladies.

Sarah and I had gone our separate ways shortly after she graduated. She ended up taking that job in Chicago after all. I don't think either of us thought we were going to marry each other—we were both too young—but still, it was painful to say good-bye. Living together gave me a preview not only of what marriage would be like, but divorce, too.

I can't say that I had ever aspired to sell copiers for a living, but I figured that trading in my apron for a suit and tie had to be a step in the right direction. People who wore suits, I'd noticed, usually got more respect. My eyebrows shot up in the way that said, "You have my undivided attention. Please, tell me more."

Once I took the bait, Jeff started to reel me in. "Most of my reps make between $30,000 and $50,000 in their first year."

My eyebrows arched higher still. I was mesmerized—borderline giddy. Fifty grand? I didn't even want to finish my lunch shift. I was tempted to resign on the spot. *Sign me up!*

But even though I could almost triple my waiter's income, I had a few concerns … minor ones, really.

For starters I didn't know *anything* about sales. I knew even less about copiers. Was it smart to enter a brand-new career field on a commission-only basis? What if I didn't sell a single copier?

Jeff saw my wheels turning.

"Tell you what," he said. "I know this is a big decision. Why don't you come along with me for a few sales calls next week? If it's not for you, no hard feelings. And if you like it, I'll teach you everything you need to know."

After tagging along on three sales calls, I was sold. I was a copier salesman.

Unbeknownst to me, the general public already had a preconception of people in my new line of work. Most copier sales reps had a reputation for being pushy hustlers who badgered their prospects until they either got the sale or got thrown out of the customer's office. Add to this aggressiveness a penchant for slicked-back hair, cheap suits, and loud, obnoxious ties, and it's easy to see why copier reps ranked only slightly above used-car salesmen on the jobs-that-the-public-views-as-extremely-cheesy scale.

Well-dressed, respectful, and professional, Jeff was an exception. He was a great mentor, and I was his new protégé. My learning curve was steep, and after a couple of months, despite my more low-pressure sales style, I had managed to sell a few copiers.

Closing a sale was more than just a financial victory. Closing a sale, no matter how small, was intoxicating … and addicting. Every deal I won was another dose of self-validation. It meant that somebody liked me, believed in me, and trusted me.

In the mirror, I saw a stunning metamorphosis from mere waiter to omnipotent salesman. Whatever the changes were, they did wonders for my dating prospects. Life could be so easy when you walked around radiating raw confidence.

◆　　◆　　◆

"Hey, Colonel, grab your jacket. I'm taking you on a sales call."

After quizzically surveying the empty office, I concluded *I* was the aforementioned colonel, and that Jeff presumably outranked me in whatever chain-of-command structure he was referencing. This was not an invitation. It was an order. I had intended to spend my day in the office, catching up on paperwork and follow-up calls, but this soldier wanted to start the day off on the right foot.

With a mock salute and a nervous smile, I replied, "Yes, sir."

I didn't feel the need, but as a precaution, I stopped in the men's room before heading out. I wasn't surprised that the pit stop turned out to be unnecessary. Aside from race-day mornings, my bowels hadn't been an issue in a couple of years. Grabbing my suit jacket, I hopped into Jeff's SUV for the trip to Longmont.

Jeff was carried away trying to fill his new sponge of a protégé with as much sales knowledge as he could during our twenty-minute drive. Today's lesson revisited the importance of "features and benefits." It worked like this:

Feature:　　　"*The 5334 copier has four different paper trays.*"

Benefit:　　　"*So, Mr. Customer, that means you will increase your productivity by saving time loading and unloading the paper trays. Isn't that great?*"

I did my best to stay focused, but my mind kept drifting off. It was Julie. She'd called again—at two in the morning. This was like the fifth time in the last two weeks, and it was really starting to piss me off.

I met Julie a few months after Sarah moved out. One day when we were walking along the Pearl Street mall, out of nowhere, she tossed it out there.

"I love you," she said in a casual way.

Caught off guard, I didn't know how to respond. So I ignored it, pretending the phrase had been neither uttered nor heard.

"Well, do you love me?" she asked.

"Julie, you know I'm crazy about you," I said. "But I'm not quite *there* yet."

"OK," she said. "But *why* don't you love me?"

I explained that after getting out of a two-year relationship with Sarah, I needed some time to make the transition. I also wanted to get to know her better. "Understand?"

"Of course I understand."

"Great, now that that's settled, let's go grab some lunch," I said.

"But *when* will you love me?"

She wasn't kidding, either. She expected a time and a date. This was nuts.

I asked her, "How can I put a timeline on my emotions?"

She apologized for jumping the gun and agreed not to pressure me.

Five minutes later, Julie restarted the sequence in an endless loop, verbatim, from the top:

"I love you." "Do you love me?" "*Why* don't you love me?" "*When* will you love me?"

And with that, our relationship plunged into an irreversible death spiral.

When I called things off, she accused me of having commitment issues. Maybe she had a point, but how could she know for sure? We'd known each other for less than three weeks.

That day on Pearl Street, two months earlier, had been our last date. Why was she still calling? How many times did you have to tell someone you weren't interested in them before they got the message? She was relentless.

Seven miles from Boulder and eight miles from Longmont, it became apparent that Julie wasn't the only problem from my past that wouldn't let go.

"But most importantly, Colonel, at the end of every sales call, you can't be timid," Jeff continued. "You have to *ask* for the sale. Remember, your business card says 'salesman.' They *expect* you to ask."

The exact sequence was a little fuzzy. One second I was looking out the Jeep's window, gazing at the Rockies' snowcapped peaks way off in the distance. I remember being only marginally aware of our more immediate surroundings—the barren, pancake-flat expanse that stretched on for miles on both sides of Highway 119.

A split second later, the tingling started. I rubbed my thumb and index finger together, feeling the light sweat seeping from my pores. It felt like race-day jitters. But what prompted my body to react like this? In my judgment, it was totally uncalled for.

Obviously I wasn't going to a race. But I wasn't even nervous or the least bit stressed. Jeff brought me along as an observer with no official responsibilities whatsoever. I had *nothing* to be concerned about. I kept telling myself this, hoping calm, logical reasoning would override the chain of events my body had erroneously set in motion.

But try as I might, I couldn't control my eyes. It didn't seem to matter that my situation was not yet urgent; my eyes darted all over the place, searching for someplace, anyplace, to ditch. Until we got to Longmont, there would be no restaurants or gas stations. No bushes or shrubs, either. Just an occasional tumbleweed blowing across the dusty flats.

I tried closing my eyes.

"I'm not boring you, am I, Colonel?"

"No, Jeff. I'm listening. I have to ask for the business."

You have nothing to be nervous about. You have nothing *to be nervous about.*

But before long, the words rang hollow. Now I did have something to be nervous about: my insides were beginning to spasm, tugging at my boxers to let me know that, like Julie, they weren't finished messing with me quite yet.

I turned my thoughts not to asking for the business, but squarely on my odds of not doing my business before we reached Longmont.

I tried to apply what I had just learned to my current situation.

Feature:	*"My bowels are touchy and ready to explode."*
Benefit:	*"So, Mr. Customer, because I'm going to spend the next fifteen minutes in your men's room, that's fifteen minutes less that you will have to spend listening to a copier salesman. Isn't that great?"*

A few minutes later, we pulled into the parking lot.

Theresa met us at the receptionist's desk and escorted us back to her cubicle. Jeff knew I had made a trip to the toilet before we left. Another trip would probably make him suspicious. Could Jeff and Theresa hear that sloshing sound? I had to speak up soon.

In a misguided approach to making people like them, salespeople tend to talk far more than they listen. Jeff was entrenched in one of his frequently recited, humorous, copier-related anecdotes. My only opportunity to interject would be during the split-second pause between this story and the next one he would surely launch into. I felt like a contestant on *Jeopardy!* waiting for the precise moment to click in with my answer.

CONTESTANT: *Alex, I'll take bathroom emergencies for $200.*

ALEX TREBEK: *A bout of this embarrassing condition can sabotage any sales opportunity.*

CONTESTANT: *What is explosive diarrhea?*

ALEX TREBEK: *CORRECT for $200!*

When my window of opportunity finally opened, I crashed through it, asking Theresa, "I'msorrybutcanI*PLEASE*useyourbathroom?"

Jeff sure hadn't seen that one coming; his eyes widened with surprise—and disappointment. I understood how he felt. It was hard to teach somebody how to become a better salesman if your star pupil was sitting in the men's room. I looked at Jeff, shrugged my shoulders, and made a beeline out of there. What a wimp I was.

When I got there, the door was locked. *Damn! Is it occupied? Or do I need a key?*

I never understood the logic behind restricting access to men's rooms. Was it a cost-saving measure designed to lower the exorbitant expense of buying the world's lowest-quality toilet paper? Or was it designed to provide employees a safe haven from undesirables—like copier salesmen?

I knocked. No answer. I knocked again, louder. No answer.

A woman walked by me, pulled out a key, and went into the ladies' room. This was bad news. I'd already been gone for a few minutes, and now I had to go and search for the key? Why hadn't Theresa told me this? I felt dumb going back to ask her now.

As if playing a demented, real-life version of *Dungeons & Dragons*, the frightened young knight snaked his way through the labyrinth of cubicles, hunching down to remain undetected by Jeff and Theresa, in his quest to wrestle his treasure from the evil Key Master—who, in this case, turned out to be a friendly receptionist who was happy to hand over the key, as long as I promised to bring it right back.

By the time I tended to my crisis and returned the key, Jeff was wrapping up the meeting. He was not impressed.

Jeff's displeasure was short lived, but I had bigger worries. I feared that my issues hadn't gone away at all—they had just been dormant all this time, waiting for the most inopportune moment to erupt again.

◆   ◆   ◆

Aside from the money, the most appealing aspect of sales was the stimulating day-to-day variety not found in office-bound professions. Each new workday brought new people to meet and new places to visit. Away from Jeff for hours at a time, I loved the freedom and autonomy.

But the downside to this grab bag of adventure into which I reached each day came in the form of unpredictability. Driving to each sales call, I had no way of knowing what to expect when I arrived, turning every workday into a gut-wrenching game of Russian roulette.

I never worried that I wouldn't be able to find a toilet. After all, where you find people, you usually find toilets. At least a third of the office buildings I visited, like the one in Longmont, had plenty of restrooms—in the same way that a bank has plenty of money: only certain people have access, and everyone else has to ask very nicely for permission to borrow it.

Knowing that every day was a leap of faith into the great unknown, I adopted some bizarre, time-consuming rituals. At the time, however, they seemed perfectly logical.

As neurotic as it sounds, I knew that if I didn't take advantage of every single opportunity to use the toilet, I would regret it later. If there was one thing I'd learned from my triathlon days, it was that there was always more toothpaste in the tube. *Always.*

I would never leave my office on the third floor without making a pit stop. After walking down the emergency stairs (I never took the elevator; what if it got stuck?), I always ducked into the lobby men's room. When I got within a mile or two of my meeting, a quick visit to a McDonald's or Circle K was obligatory. It wasn't unheard of to stop again if another, closer opportunity presented itself.

A decade later, *Fear Factor* would become one of the most popular reality TV shows. In each episode, a $50,000 prize would entice contestants to face and overcome their greatest fears. Whether the challenge was eating a bucket of beetles or being placed in a worm-packed coffin, the show would reveal exactly how far people were willing to go for the right amount of money. Of course, in 1994 I was playing my own version of *Fear Factor*—five days a week, for twelve long months. Was I willing to endure my daily fear of crapping my pants during a sales call in exchange for $50,000?

I certainly had no intention of going back to waiting tables.

◆　　◆　　◆

If there's one thing that salespeople love, it's an inbound lead.

A rare occurrence, especially in the copier business, an inbound lead is a gift from above. It means some masochist in your territory has *voluntarily* picked up the phone and *willingly* requested that a sales rep visit his office to talk about copiers. It's akin to requesting a home visit from a Jehovah's Witness. I'd been working for Jeff for almost a year when I received the mother of all inbound leads.

Bottomless Pit, a local, all-you-can-eat barbecue chain, was expanding across the western states. To handle all the paperwork, they needed not one, but *two* robust copiers. The kind of copiers with all the bells and whistles. The kind of copiers that cost a fortune. The kind of copiers that come with huge commission checks.

From the moment I set foot in the Bottomless Pit headquarters for our first meeting, I had a great feeling about this deal. Their men's room was the stuff of daydreams. Located near the elevators, just down the hall from the reception area and well beyond earshot of their offices and meeting rooms, it boasted ten glistening stalls, all in a row. And best of all, it was open to everyone—no key required. It was odd, but just knowing that I would have access to such a facility made every meeting with Bottomless Pit a walk in the park.

The big deals usually took longer to close. After two months of going back and forth, the folks at Bottomless Pit liked our pricing, they liked us, and they liked our copiers. Only one major box needed to be checked: the demo.

Even though this was technically my deal, Jeff wanted to help coach his not-fully-experienced rep from the sidelines. I loved the arrangement: he would help me close the deal and strengthen my sales skills, and I would get the commission.

"OK, Colonel, this is great," Jeff said. "We're in the home stretch, and this deal is ours to lose. We've got to finish strong on this one. The whole deal is riding on a successful demo. If we pull off a good one, we're both going to be doing the 'I'm so happy' dance. Got it?"

Jeff was the type of guy who didn't leave anything to chance, especially when it came to huge opportunities like this. He got worked up as he brainstormed what we could do to wow Susan, the purchasing manager at Bottomless Pit who would come to Denver to evaluate our demo.

As if I needed any further motivation, Jeff pulled out his calculator, typed in a stream of numbers, and showed me exactly how big my commission check would be. As I recall, the figure was in the neighborhood of $10,000—attention-getting, to say the least. I was on board.

"First, make sure you reserve the demo room downtown," Jeff instructed.

"Of course. I'll do it today," I replied.

"Then, make sure you put a service call in on the demo machine. We need to have that 5385 in top form, firing on all cylinders. Got it?"

"A service call. Yes, I'll make sure to place that call today," I enthusiastically assured him. After writing down his instructions, I daydreamed about what I would do with my earnings. *Pay off my credit card debt ... drink a lot of margaritas ... maybe buy a new suit ... I could always use a bigger TV ... put a deposit down on a Winnebago, so I can drive to all my sales calls with my own toilet.*

"Colonel, I got it. You absolutely have to go that extra mile and roll out the red carpet for Susan. You need to call her and tell her that you'll pick her up in Boulder, drive her to Denver, do the demo, and then drive her back to her office. Door-to-door chauffeur service. OK?"

What? How did you come up with this crazy idea? No, not OK. Boulder to Denver was about a forty-minute drive. I visualized getting stuck in traffic with Susan riding shotgun in my car. The whole point of this exercise was to get her to like me so she'd do business with me. Jeff had clearly chosen the wrong man for this mission.

"Jeff, that's a great idea. The only problem is that I don't think she'll be impressed riding in my small, beat-up VW. My air-conditioning doesn't even work. I'm sure she's probably expecting to drive herself down there anyway." *That should do the trick. How can he argue with that?*

Jeff didn't even pause to process my argument. "Look, take my car if you want, but just get her down there."

I must have telegraphed my disappointment. Jeff stared at me, dumbfounded.

"Why am I getting the feeling you don't think this is a good idea? I'm trying to help you win this deal. Any salesman in his right mind would die for the chance to spend a few hours of captive face time with their biggest prospect. Why aren't you jumping all over this?"

He thought I wasn't willing to go the extra mile to win the deal. I wanted to tell him that I was doing everything in my power not to *lose* the deal.

I reconsidered his suggestion, trying to envision a panic-free drive with Susan. It *was* a good idea, and I wished that I could carry it out.

But each time I ran it through my head, my mind and bowels conspired to paint one horrific vision after another.

Would I be willing to risk disaster for the chance to earn $10,000? I had my answer: no way. I clung to the hope that we could still somehow win the business without offering lavish door-to-door transportation.

Though it had been phrased as a suggestion, Jeff's plan was an order. Disobeying an order, I feared, could result in a court-martial. I was neither lazy nor subordinate, and I needed to find a way to appease Jeff and still cash the $10,000 commission check. He was waiting for my answer.

"Jeff, I hear what you're saying, and I think it's a good idea. To tell you the truth, I'm nervous that I might run out of things to say or maybe even say the *wrong* thing. I just don't want to blow this."

Jeff looked disappointed but not furious. "Well, Colonel, it's your deal, and it's your decision. If I were in your shoes, I wouldn't let this opportunity slip away. But … it probably won't prevent us from winning. Let's hope for the best and make sure we kick ass at the demo. It has to be perfect, understand?"

It wasn't the best outcome, but I was still in the game. Not wanting to take any more chances, I placed the service call, reserved the demo room for the following Thursday, and crossed my fingers.

When the big day arrived, I drove down to Denver early to make sure our demo copier was working flawlessly. I put the massive 5385 through its paces by testing all of its capabilities: reduction, enlargement, collating, sorting, stapling, color highlighting, and automatic document feeding. I confirmed it was full of toner and well stocked with paper. Check, check, check. All systems go. Jeff arrived a few minutes later to help me run the demo.

Susan arrived right on schedule. After saying hello and welcoming her, I ran to the men's room to put my digestive tract through all of *its* paces. Once the demo started, I would have no time for a trip to the toilet. At this point, I was sure Jeff would fire me for such an ill-timed move. Like the reliable 5385, my colon rapidly spit out several duplicates of its morning's work. Check, check, check. All systems go.

The first twenty minutes of the demonstration went according to plan. No misfires. No paper jams. No error codes. Reliability in action. It was impressive to watch.

The copier sales community has a term to describe when a copier malfunctions in dramatic fashion in front of a sales prospect: throwing up. Near the end of the demo, our 5385 threw up in a big way. Attempting to reproduce an original 11 x 17 color poster color poster that Susan had brought along, the 5385 not only jammed in two separate paper trays, but also violently mangled, then ejected, Susan's original document. It was as if we had just watched a grizzly bear storm into the office, then savagely devour a defenseless kitten and spit out the bones.

Everybody was in shock. Had we really just seen that? Susan was horrified. Jeff was furious. In all likelihood, I was unemployed.

Surprisingly, despite our copier's brutal mauling of her poster, Susan recommended that Bottomless Pit buy our copiers anyway. And I deposited a large check into my bank account. If only the story ended there.

Even though we got the sale, Jeff lost confidence in me. He had made it clear to me that the demo needed to go perfectly. Clearly it hadn't. Jeff didn't blame me for the 5385 throwing up, but he correctly pointed out that by not chauffeuring Susan to and from the demo, I had jeopardized the deal. With that, the Colonel was dishonorably discharged, putting an end to my short career in copier sales.

I'd gotten used to being rejected by clients, but the sting of being rejected by Jeff—my mentor, my coach, my friend—sent my confidence into a tailspin. I spent the next two weeks in a fog of depression where I drank way too much tequila, slept well into the afternoon, and showered only sporadically. I was a mess.

I put off calling my mom. I'd have to come up with a pretty creative story to explain this turn of events. I didn't have the energy.

If I couldn't hold down a job selling copiers, what would my future hold? What career field would grant me unrestricted access to a men's room and also give me the chance to earn a comfortable living? Without much in the way of savings, I had to figure it out soon.

Hell on Wheels

When it came to the financial industry, I was clueless. Even though initial public offerings, technology stocks, NASDAQ, and mutual funds were creating countless new millionaires each day, they were unfamiliar terms that meant nothing to me. Despite my obvious lack of qualifications, I inexplicably stumbled onto my dream job with Robertson Stephens, a prominent investment bank that took start-up technology companies public more frequently than I visited the men's room.

I spent each day working on the twenty-fifth floor of the Bank of America building, high above the thick morning fog and the hustle and bustle of the fast-paced city below. From my desk, I enjoyed a postcard vista of San Francisco: Telegraph Hill, Coit Tower, Alcatraz, and, in the distance, the Golden Gate Bridge. My younger sister, Lisa, lived nearby and had offered to help me follow in her professional footsteps in the investment business.

My mom was thrilled. She just couldn't wait for the next Greenwich cocktail party to boast about my achievements. She'd endured fours years of "my son the aspiring triathlete and part-time waiter." She had barely tolerated "my son the copier salesman." This was the moment she had been waiting for.

"Tim, my oldest, lives in San Francisco now," she would toss out, withholding the nature of my occupation in a calculated attempt to invite a follow-up query. "Oh, what does he do for a living? Tim is in investment banking," she would proclaim with pride.

This, of course, was stretching the hell out of the truth. My employer was an investment bank. I, however, worked for a division of the firm that managed and sold mutual funds.

What I soon learned was that within the broad world of finance and investment banking, selling mutual funds was on par with selling copiers. I didn't analyze the market. I didn't recommend stocks. I didn't wager the firm's capital on promising new start-up technology companies.

No, I sold mutual funds to investors. Like a waiter reciting the daily lunch specials, I tried to entice the masses of individual investors to buy what was hot and tasty each day. But to the layperson (and to me, before I knew what I was talking about), it seemed like a glamorous Wall Street career. It didn't matter how many times I tried to set them straight; in my family's eyes, I was a hotshot investment banker. "Hell on wheels," my grandmother had said.

Allan was the manager of the sales team and a former football player. He liked to hire athletes because they brought a competitive, hard-charging attitude to his team. If the candidate also happened to have sales experience, so much the better.

Glancing at my accomplishments on a thirty-two-pound sheet of ivory stationery, it would be hard for Allan *not* to like what he saw *Triathlete, copier-sales experience, studied economics.* The problem with résumés, of course, was that they could be dangerously misleading, letting employers see only what they wanted to see. Allan had no way of knowing what had transpired back in Colorado. It seemed a wise omission.

During our interview, I had cranked the old first-impression machine into high gear. From where Allan sat, I looked like a successful salesman, sounded like a successful salesman, and—at the moment anyway—even smelled like a successful salesman.

Investment people often use the terms "upside" and "downside" to refer to the pros and cons of any given situation. I had managed to stumble onto a job that offered plenty of the former.

My new employer was going to teach me everything I needed to know about mutual funds and pay me to learn about this exciting industry. I had the potential to earn two or three times more than I ever had, which was a good thing because living and dating in San Francisco was beyond expensive.

I was relieved to learn that all my sales calls would be exactly that—calls, as in phone calls. Day in and day out, my work environment would never change. Sure, I was sacrificing the autonomy I'd enjoyed while selling copiers, but knowing that the men's room would always be unlocked and in the same place every day was enormously comforting. But the upside didn't end there. Working in the investment business carried far more prestige with San Francisco's women than selling copiers.

This job did have some downside. Twelve-hour workdays were the rule rather than the exception. But working long hours turned out to be a positive thing because it kept me from spending money I didn't yet have. Until I received my year-end bonus check eight months later, it would be challenging to live within my means on my starting salary of $25,000. Out of necessity, my budgeting efforts included sharing an apartment with a pothead roommate above a noisy karaoke bar, buying five-gallon vats of peanut butter and jelly at Costco, and taking public transportation to work.

I lived three hilly miles from my downtown office—too far to walk and, with the high cost of parking in my office building, too costly to drive. In my new neighborhood, half of the residents had jobs in the technology industry, and the other half worked in the investment business. Consequently half drove their BMWs or Porsches down toward Silicon Valley each morning while half left their four-wheeled status symbols at home and boarded the 30X.

The 30X is short for the San Francisco Muni #30 express bus line. It ferries throngs of attractive, well-groomed, pleasantly scented, young professionals from the yuppie-filled Marina District to the Financial District. I lived across Lombard Street in nearby Cow Hollow, but the Marina was the closest place to catch the bus. Compared to the price of public parking downtown, the bus's $1 fare was a bargain; and even factoring in the stops, the entire commute usually only lasted about fifteen minutes. If you worked downtown, riding the 30X was a no-brainer.

I remember being excited about my first day. Dressed in my navy blue suit, red tie, and well-shined loafers, I fit right in with the other fifteen financial types waiting for the 30X on Chestnut Street.

After feeding my crisp $1 bill into the fare slot, I staked out a standing position near the rear door of the nearly filled coach. I felt as if I had mistakenly walked into a photo shoot for a J. Crew or a Brooks Brothers catalog. While everybody looked all-American, this group of young, well-dressed, and mostly white commuters was far from what I'd call a representative slice of America. At each of the remaining five stops along Chestnut Street, an endless stream of these perfect-looking, Stepford commuters piled in.

After picking up its final passenger, our bus began the one-mile express leg of our trip downtown. Within three or four minutes, I figured, I would be walking into my new office for my first day of work.

Twenty minutes later, and less than a half mile from my downtown destination, rush-hour traffic had trapped us inside the Broadway tunnel. People began to glance down at their Rolex watches and impatiently tap their Gucci-clad feet. The yuppies were growing restless.

Traffic showed no signs of moving, but my bowels were beginning to. Knowing that they'd already performed admirably this morning provided little comfort. As the legal disclaimer that appears in mutual fund advertisements says, past performance is no guarantee of future performance.

As I fretfully pondered whether this ride would ultimately end in disaster for me, I revisited a long-standing question: if I did have an accident, exactly how obvious would it be? My only reference point was an unpleasant high-school memory that my subconscious was now dredging to the surface.

After a ski race in northern New Jersey, twelve of us were returning to campus in the school's van. Three hours earlier, when we'd arrived

at the mountain, I'd found out too late that the lodge was closed …
and the race shack had no toilet. I got caught in the worst way: with
my pants up. Using fresh snow and my soon-to-be-discarded long
underwear, I'd cleaned myself to the best of my ability. A few hours
later, and only five minutes into our return trip back to school, Kendall, sitting to my immediate left, wasn't happy.

He took a deep breath and yanked his turtleneck collar well above
his nose. "Oh my God, that is so uncool. Who did that?"

Nobody said anything. The minutes passed, and Kendall's turtleneck eventually descended from his face. The crisis seemed to be over.

Moments later, after another reluctant sniff, Kendall's tone
became more threatening. "Damn it, somebody dropped another one!
Who was it?"

Silence. Who in their right mind would confess to such a crime?
Certainly not me. I couldn't believe how long my luck had already
lasted. Could he possibly continue to think somebody was merely
passing gas?

Kendall again hoisted his turtleneck and raised his voice. "Who the
hell *keeps* doing that?" His questions were not born out of curiosity, as
if merely identifying the odor's source would solve some brainteaser
he was working on. He was on a warpath. This was about inflicting
physical retribution, pure and simple.

When it became clear that no confession would be forthcoming,
Kendall eventually put two and two together. "Wait a minute … I
think somebody crapped his pants!"

I spent the rest of the ride with my Walkman on and my eyes
closed, trying to give the appearance of guiltless slumber. Nobody
ever fingered me as the culprit.

Standing on the bus that day, I still wondered exactly how Kendall
made that leap from gas to solid. Did one smell distinctly different
than the other? Or was it the stench's refusal to dissipate? The answer
had direct relevance for me.

When I looked around, I saw that more than a few of these young
professionals came across as self-absorbed and arrogant. Their smug atti-

tudes seemed to say, "*My* shit doesn't stink." Maybe so, but mine sure did—a fact that I hoped these people would never find out firsthand.

Why should I care about what a busload of total strangers thought of me?

I cared because these people were strangers only because I had not been introduced to them *yet*. We all lived in the same small part of town, shopped at the same stores, and drank at the same bars. We also worked in the same industry, where everyone seemed to know one another. In all likelihood, I would eventually find myself either working with some of them or maybe even asking them for a job.

Equally important, having recently moved to town, I didn't yet have any dating prospects. The bus was packed with attractive, young, professional women. One of the tenets of sound investing is not putting all your eggs in one basket. Being known as the guy who "lost it" on the 30X would be more than humiliating. It would render me a professional and social leper.

I had to get away from these people. I had to get off this bus.

"Excuse me, please," I said, reaching for my lifeline—the semislack plastic cord hanging above the windows.

"What are you *doing?*" asked the man whose *Wall Street Journal* I had accidentally knocked down.

"Sorry about that," I said. "I'm late. I'm going to get off and walk." I yanked the cord twice to make sure the driver noticed. I heard the bell ring twice. So did everybody else. But the doors remained closed. As I reached to tug the cord again, I noticed that I was on center stage.

My friend with the *Wall Street Journal* was kind enough to bring the oblivious rookie up to speed. "What are you thinking? You can't get off before Montgomery. It's an *express* bus."

"But we're not even moving," I protested. "Do they expect us to just *sit* here?"

Returning his eyes to the *Journal*, he said, "Yeah, pretty much." He said it as if being trapped against your will in an overcrowded bus in a dark tunnel was not a grave injustice on par with a violation of the Geneva Convention, but rather something of a nonevent. Who knew how much longer it would be before the bus left the tunnel and pulled onto Montgomery Street? I was seething over my involuntary confinement.

My feeling of helplessness briefly gave way to my raw fury. I wanted to hit somebody. I wanted to *kill* somebody. This was criminal!

Preoccupied with retribution, I almost didn't realize the bus had begun to roll forward. The wheels were turning slowly, but we were at least moving. Motion—any motion—was progress. Motion was hope. Motion meant that the terror wasn't going to last forever.

It wasn't long before rays of natural light beamed through the bus's windshield. Seconds later, the tops of the tall, silver towers of the Bay Bridge, shimmering beneath the morning sun, came into view. After a momentary tap on the brakes, the wheels started to roll once again. Seeing the acres of drying laundry that hung perpetually from Chinatown's fire escapes like ornaments from a Charlie Brown Christmas tree, I knew that I had survived the Broadway tunnel and was now just around the corner from Montgomery Street.

In reality how frequently did the 30X get stuck inside the Broadway tunnel? I had no idea. And in my mind, the answer didn't matter. Even if something like this happened only once every year, that would be too often. After only one ride, I had completed my analysis. Riding this bus carried far too much downside.

On my first day on the job, I spent twelve hours focused not on learning about mutual funds and how to sell them, but on finding a new way to get to and from the office. Beginning that evening, I started riding the 41 Union, which, unlike the 30X, was a local route that made stops on every other block and bypassed the Broadway tunnel altogether. It was a convenient solution while it lasted, but after arriving noticeably late to work three times in a two-week period, I had run out of affordable, reliable, bowel-friendly ways to get to work. Something had to give.

◆   ◆   ◆

"Hey, Tim, what kind of car do you drive?" asked Mike, a co-worker who sat at the next desk and lived a few blocks down the street from me.

"A Volkswagen," I said, careful not to divulge too much information until I knew where this line of questioning was headed.

"Is it a GTI by any chance?" he asked.

"As a matter of fact, it is."

"Orange?" he asked.

"*Orange?* No. Who would buy an orange car?" I said. Although ten years of sunlight had faded the paint to where it might appear light orange, my car was in fact red. "Why? Are you testing out your psychic abilities?"

"No, nothing like that," Mike said. "I saw a guy who looked exactly like you drive by while I was waiting for the 30X this morning."

"Really?" I asked.

"Yeah, but then I wondered why you would pay for parking instead of taking the bus. It didn't make sense."

"Yeah, why would I do that? That's crazy."

"I knew it couldn't have been you because you would have stopped and given me a ride, right?"

"Of course I would have," I assured him. "*If* I drove to work ... but I don't."

How could I have been so sloppy? I nearly jeopardized the whole operation. That was the last thing I needed: someone else in the car with me. Beginning the next morning, I drove along a different route, making sure to steer well clear of Chestnut Street.

The parking garage in the Bank of America building charged an egregious sum of $28 a day, a fee I would never have paid even if I could have afforded to. But only four blocks away, I found another garage that charged only $18, which was still pricey but far more reasonable. I soon figured out the reason for this $10 price discrepancy: if you didn't have the cardiovascular capacity of a mountain goat, you would have to pay a cabbie close to that amount to carry you up those four nearly vertical blocks of California Street that formed the face of Nob Hill to get to the garage. It had been almost two years since my last triathlon, and each strenuous ascent left me with cramped calves and a sweat-soaked button-down shirt.

Compared to the bus, I was paying an extra $16 each day, five days a week, just to get to and from the office. I felt like I was being extorted by the mob. I couldn't afford to pay for this "insurance," but I also couldn't afford not to. *Hey pal, look, if you don't pay us eighty bucks each week, it's possible something could, you know, "happen" to your ass, if you know what we're saying.* Capiche?

San Francisco was expensive enough in its own right. The added cost of accommodating my body's gastrointestinal whims made it even tougher to live within my means.

Paraphrasing a Chinese proverb, it's a foolish man who knows the cost of everything but the value of nothing. The cost of daily parking was exorbitant, but the value was undeniable. The added expense of driving to work assured me an anxiety-free way of getting to and from an anxiety-free work environment. Compared to the alternative, I considered this money well spent.

◆   ◆   ◆

Fourteen months after moving to San Francisco, it was clear to me that getting fired by Jeff had been a blessing in disguise. My new life in San Francisco had become everything I could have hoped for—and then some. I even managed to find myself in a relationship. For the first time in years, I was beginning to believe that I could have it all.

Examining the recent trends, my mom couldn't help but work herself up into a frenzied lather. First a great career … and now a girl-friend. Could a daughter-in-law and a grandchild be far behind? She wanted to hear all about this young woman I was so smitten with. How had we met?

"Tim, don't you mean a mutual *friend?*" she asked, assuming I had misspoken.

"No," I assured her. "We met through a mutual *fund.*"

Technically I met Cynthia through a mutual *friend* with whom I sold mutual *funds*. But I liked telling it this way because I loved that brief but delightful split second of head-scratching awkwardness. *Is this guy that stupid?*

Cynthia was a petite twenty-six-year-old with dark brown hair and the bluest eyes I'd ever seen. She had a good job in software sales. Though serious about her career, Cynthia also had a silly, goofy side. Carefree and spontaneous, she was the perfect counterbalance for me. As quickly as I hit the brakes, Cynthia stomped on the gas. My default response to trying new things was increasingly becoming either "No" or "Why?" Cynthia, on the other hand, navigated her way through life with one "Fuck, yeah" or "Why the hell not?" after another.

"I can't wait to meet her," my mom said. "And how about work? Is everything still going well?"

"Couldn't be better, Mom. Couldn't be better."

I wasn't lying. Back at the office, I had become reasonably successful at selling mutual funds. In fairness this was not especially difficult to do. With our mutual funds boasting eye-popping, 90 percent annual returns, my job was about as challenging as selling winning Powerball tickets in a trailer park: right place, right time.

Because my performance was at least on par with that of my peers, I was surprised when I was summoned to Allan's office. What had I done wrong? Was I going to be fired for the second time in two years? My mom might never recover.

"Tim, I'd like you to consider taking a new position in our financial advisor group," Allan said. "This is a chance for you to make a lot more money than you're making now."

His offer to promote me came completely out of the blue. Did he say *a lot* more money? *OK, Allan, I'm still listening.*

"You would be calling on financial advisors in our southeast territory. That's everything from Virginia to Florida and over to Louisiana."

It sounded perfect. I'd gone to college in the South and was comfortable dealing with Southerners. Instead of calling on emotional individual investors, I would be calling on sophisticated investment professionals. And I'd be making *a lot* more money—certainly enough to cover my parking costs. And all from the comfort of my desk overlooking San Francisco Bay. *Where do I sign up?*

"Of course, we'll give you an expense account to cover your entertainment and travel costs."

Whoa! Travel? What travel? What's he talking about? Why would I need an expense account to make calls?

Allan explained that I would have to fly to the East Coast every other week for these sales calls (sales "voyages" would be more accurate). Not only would I be thrown back into the torturous and unnerving shell game of guessing the location of the nearest accessible toilet, but I also would face the additional stress of flying—the one thing I dreaded more than riding the 30X. This was not the type of promotion I wanted.

If I couldn't even come up with a good reason for not riding the bus to work, how on earth would I explain my rationale for not accepting this dream promotion? Unlike Jeff, Allan still believed in me and expected great things from me. I was torn between the loyalty I owed him and my fierce aversion to what would be my new professional life.

Allan suggested that I fly out to a three-day conference for financial advisors in Denver the following week. This trip, he said, would give me a chance to try my new position on for size and see if it fit. I made my reservations and confirmed an aisle seat in the last row, near the lavatory.

I slept very little the night before my trip. When I wasn't worrying about my big career decision or my morning flight to Denver, I was kept awake by a pronunciation-challenged singer painfully belting out tunes in the karaoke bar beneath my bedroom. I'm still not sure which was more agonizing: the thought of soiling my pants in midflight or suffering through his torturous rendition of the Eagles classic, "Despe*wado*."

It had been several months since I'd last driven to San Francisco International Airport, and I had forgotten just how slow rush hour had become. I jumped in my beat-up VW and joined the tightly packed conga line of barely moving, high-performance vehicles that stretched from my doorstep to San Jose sixty miles away.

I pulled into SFO's long-term parking lot and waited for the shuttle bus to the terminal. From my parking spot, I saw something terrifying: out on the runway, no fewer than fifteen jets were backed up awaiting takeoff. Gridlock, it seemed, was everywhere.

Try as I might, I could not stop thinking about all those jets waiting in line. It was clear the planes at the back weren't getting into the air anytime in the next thirty or forty minutes. And thanks to the FAA's safety regulations, all the passengers sitting out there in those jam-packed planes wouldn't be getting out of their seats—for any reason—anytime soon, either. Flight attendants, I knew from personal experience, were adamant about enforcing that rule.

As another jet taxied toward the end of the line, I no longer saw a plane. I saw the 30X ... with wings.

Allowing myself to indulge in such terrifying thoughts came with a physical price. Without my consent, the process had been set in motion. With the shuttle bus nowhere in sight, I was forced to put my imagination into high gear.

TV's problem solver extraordinaire, MacGyver, always saved the day by combining a set of perfectly ill-suited resources with a whole lot of ingenuity. My immediate resources consisted of a Hefty trash bag from my trunk, two mutual fund prospectuses from my briefcase, and the backseat of my VW hatchback.

Talk about a challenging morning. I'd endured an abysmally typical rush hour, temporarily converted my car into a makeshift toilet, braved a forty-minute, butt-cheek-clenching tour of the tarmac before takeoff, and I still hadn't gotten to work yet.

Only a week earlier, I finally had everything in my life exactly as I wanted it. It was perfect. Now that I glimpsed my future, I hated it. I couldn't embrace it, but I felt obligated to accept it.

All I wanted was to stay in my new city with my new girlfriend and my old job.

Dam!

I was ready.

Two months shy of my thirtieth birthday, I'd had enough of the variety and excitement. I yearned for a life of stability and predictability. I craved the unwavering support that could come only from a trusted partner—a partner I could count on to help get me through good times and bad. So, on a foggy afternoon in July of 1996, I took the plunge and walked down the aisle for the first time.

The Walgreens employees called it Aisle Four. For me it would be forever known as the aisle of embarrassing products. Not by coincidence, Aisle Four was rarely crowded. I suspected I wasn't the only person who circled the aisle's entrance in a holding pattern, waiting for the opportunity to fill my basket under a blanket of anonymity. In those aisles where shampoo or batteries are sold, eye contact between customers was acceptable. But not here.

My new job would subject me to a biweekly barrage of commuting traffic, airport security lines, runway gridlock, connecting flights, and office buildings that had only a one-in-three chance of having unlocked toilets. Any *one* of these threats carried the potential to send my bowels into instantaneous revolt. Taken together, the whole was far greater than the sum of my anxieties. Unless I wanted to live every other week in absolute terror, I needed to be proactive. I needed to go on offense.

Years later, I would look back and recognize this moment as one of many times when the wise course of action would have been to visit a doctor. Back then, however, I'd convinced myself I was the only person on the face of the earth with this peculiar combination of mental and physical issues. Even if I wanted to, how would I begin to explain my unusual—not to mention embarrassing—symptoms? And who exactly would I explain them to? A primary-care physician? A psychiatrist? A proctologist? No thanks.

So instead, applying a modicum of intrinsic male logic, I crafted a solution that was as ingenious as it was straightforward. To keep my gastrointestinal tract from spilling its contents all over my life, I would head down to the store, pick up some supplies, and build a dam.

The first offerings in this gauntlet of personal products were relatively innocuous: condoms and a wide assortment of sexual lubricants. In my teenage years, buying "rubbers" had been a face-reddening rite of passage. How times have changed. These days, thanks to Dr. Ruth and former Surgeon General Jocelyn Elders, people who *don't* buy condoms and practice safe sex are castigated.

Next stop: feminine products. On more than one occasion, I had been tasked with picking up a box of Tampax. Granted, it wasn't as mindlessly comfortable as buying a can of shaving cream, but it was nothing to dread, either. It wasn't as if anybody in their right mind would think they were for me.

Scanning farther down the aisle, my eyes came to a widened halt. The product sitting on the shelf before me was more than embarrassing. It was a terrifying glimpse into how bad my condition could potentially become. Thirty-year-olds like me didn't live in retirement communities in Del Ray Beach, Florida. They didn't drive Cadillacs. And they sure as hell didn't wear Depends adult diapers.

As my tour continued, I moved from a product I *hoped* I would never need to a product I *knew* I'd never need. I felt a twinge of jealousy toward people who needed Ex-Lax. *Lucky bastards!*

At last, after zipping past the Gas-X and Preparation H, I arrived at the antidiarrheal medications.

My mom had given me Pepto-Bismol for my occasional bouts of childhood diarrhea and nausea. Seeing the radioactive-looking pink liquid through the transparent bottle made me recall the high price I'd paid for faking stomachaches to ditch school. My eyes winced and my mouth puckered as my taste buds relived the unique medicine flavor.

Imodium was a product I'd heard of but had not yet tried. "Maximum Strength!" the label exclaimed. Also printed in a billboard-sized font for the entire world to see was "Anti-Diarrheal." And just in case that didn't quite spell things out, an additional line of oversized copy offered further clarification: "Controls the symptoms of diarrhea."

Well, nobody could mistake what this stuff was for. Like a condom, Imodium has but one use. The mere possession of this product announces to one and all, "Hey, keep your distance, and nobody gets hurt."

That's why I chose Pepto-Bismol. Any onlookers who might be interested in speculating on the nature of my ailment (I was convinced they all were) faced a multiple-choice guessing game, with the odds of winning being exactly one in five. In small, subtle print, the label promised temporary relief for heartburn, indigestion, upset stomach, nausea, and diarrhea.

I could chug this stuff in plain view for all to see, and I would have but a 20 percent chance of being charged with diarrhea. Expecting to encounter the occasional suspicious look, I prepared a well-rehearsed response: place both palms over my left breast, nod to acknowledge the obvious, and whisper, "Heartburn."

Because I couldn't find the elixir that specifically promised to halt the endless procession of rogue stools sprinting from my body whenever I wasn't near a bathroom, I figured Pepto was my best chance. I was working on a hunch.

Although I didn't always have classic diarrhea symptoms, my theory—and hope—was that Pepto would provide an additional layer of slowing, or blocking, whatever my body's starting point. With a few swigs of Pepto, those with diarrhea would become regular; the already regular would become constipated; and the already constipated, I imagined, would ... well, let's just say spontaneous human combustion might not have been out of the question.

Supplies in hand, I was eager to get home and start building the dam.

◆   ◆   ◆

Cynthia couldn't sit still. "Don't make any plans for next weekend. We're getting out of the city."

"We are?" I asked. "Why?"

"So we can celebrate your big promotion," Cynthia said.

"Where are we going?"

"Carmel!" she said. Like a mother on Christmas morning who has just given her son the Big Wheel he'd always wanted, she waited for the tears of unbridled joy to stream down my face. "Surprised?"

"Surprised?" I repeated. "Believe me, you have no idea how surprised I am."

Without my knowledge or consent, Cynthia had taken the liberty of planning all the details of our weekend getaway, including making a reservation at a bed and breakfast.

"Guess what? Our room has a fireplace *and* a Jacuzzi." Without pausing for a single breath, Cynthia went on, "I'll bring my CDs and my candles ... *lots* of candles! Oh, bring your khakis, a button-down, and a sport coat, so we can go out for a fancy dinner. Ocean Avenue has lots of quaint restaurants and bistros. I've been bottled up in the city way too long. I can't wait to take my shoes off and walk on the beach. The B&B isn't far from the water, so we can walk down. You're not going to believe how amazing the sunsets are. It's going to be such a fun weekend. I am so psyched!"

My reaction was somewhat different.

It should come as no surprise that I'd never once been to Carmel, despite its proximity to San Francisco. I didn't have a clue as to how we'd get there. I assumed we'd take 101 South for a while, but at some point, we'd have to head west, toward the ocean. What kind of roads would those be? Would they have places to stop? What if they didn't? Carmel was a popular tourist spot—would we run into a lot of traffic? And if so, for how long? Would there be a public toilet at the beach? What about the "quaint" restaurants Cynthia described? Quaint places tend to be small places, and small places often have only one bathroom. What if I made a dash for the one toilet, only to find it occupied? Would I risk waiting it out or leave the restaurant to search for an alternate toilet?

So many uninvited thoughts careened through my brain, all in the split second after Cynthia uttered "Carmel."

On Friday afternoon, Cynthia and I loaded up her company-issued Ford Taurus. She was bouncing up and down, jittery from the anticipation of our romantic weekend.

"Are you excited?" she asked.

"Don't I look excited?" I asked.

"Honestly? No, not really," she said, her smile disappearing.

"I'm sorry. I *am* excited. I'm just preoccupied with work and my new job," I said, hoping that playing the clichéd *work is stressing me out* card would buy me a little latitude—which it did.

"I understand you're nervous," she said. "But I think you're worrying about nothing. I have a feeling you're going to kick ass, and you'll probably even get promoted again."

She leaned over, gave me a kiss, and handed me the keys.

For reasons unknown, navigating through the city to the freeway on-ramp was a breeze. Ordinarily the streets running through the industrialized South of Market area were backed up before you could even see the entrance to 101 South, but we were able to race down Tenth Street unimpeded. In no time, we were out of San Francisco and barreling south.

As we blew past the airport, I couldn't help but notice the jets backed up for takeoff. Nine, I counted—a sobering reminder of what lay in store for me the week after next. At eighty miles per hour, it wasn't long before we passed Palo Alto. As we closed in on San Jose, we were nearing uncharted territory for me. Because San Jose was the farthest south I'd ever ventured, I had no idea what horrors and obstacles might lay on the other side. I felt like Christopher Columbus sailing toward what might be the edge of the earth.

Not only, as the famous song once asked, did I "know the *way* to San Jose," but thanks to a series of highway markers, I now knew the exact distance, too.

SAN JOSE 10 MILES

Since my goal had been to have the dam up and running by the time we left for Carmel, I'd started to hit the pink stuff three days earlier, on Tuesday. By day's end, the recommended dose of two tablespoons had made no impact whatsoever. Suspecting that my stocky physical frame might have a higher tolerance for this stuff, I'd erred on the side of overdoing it. Doubling my dose, I sought that middle ground between being sufficiently backed up and the more severe possibility of exploding into flames.

SAN JOSE 7 MILES

At work on Wednesday, the anticipation of our little weekend getaway had forced me to make eight separate trips to the men's room. It seemed four tablespoons of Pepto the night before, and four more when I'd woken up in the morning, had still been no match for the relentless forces of nature. Coming home that night and seeing the bottle still half full, I'd chugged it all—every last drop. A few hours later, I'd walked back over to Walgreens, and back down the aisle, for another bottle. The dam still needed to be stronger.

SAN JOSE 5 MILES

By Thursday night, I had begun to chug the stuff around the clock. My overconsumption meant still more trips to Walgreens and more trips down the aisle. I suppose I could have gone to Costco, but I couldn't get comfortable with the image of pushing a shopping cart filled with a five-gallon drum of Pepto-Bismol through the aisles.

"Is that all for you, sir?" the cashier would ask. Women behind me in line would raise their eyebrows, prompting my chest-clutching, lip-synched reply: "Heartburn."

The dam was working, but not at full strength, I feared.

SAN JOSE CITY LIMITS

What awaited me on the other side of the city limits? Anything seemed possible. In the face of such uncertainty and danger, history's great explorers found the courage to press on.

Not me.

"I'm thirsty," I told Cynthia. "Do you mind if we make a stop?"

"Fine by me. We're in no hurry."

I dashed into a minimart near downtown San Jose, paid $1.50 for a bottle of water I did not want, shelled out $4 for a small bottle of Pepto I *did* want, and helped myself to the men's room. The dam was still not at full strength. I guzzled close to half the pink bottle, threw the rest away (I couldn't take it with me), and walked back to the car.

Stopping when I did turned out to be a smart move. The situation started getting bad once we passed San Jose and the road narrowed from three lanes to two—a clear announcement that we were headed away from civilization and toward someplace more desolate. It wasn't an immediate shift, but little by little, I saw fewer and fewer exits and service stations. It wouldn't be long before we would have to say good-bye to 101 and whatever remaining amenities it offered.

We passed a sign promising fuel, food, and lodging at the Gilroy exit, two miles up the road.

"I'm hungry. Do you mind if we make another stop?"

Cynthia was surprised, but not quite annoyed. "We'll be there in an hour. You can't wait?"

"No, I don't think so. Didn't you say we're not in a hurry?"

"I guess you're right. Go ahead and stop if you want to."

I repeated the exact same drill I'd performed thirty minutes earlier in San Jose, only this time replacing the unnecessary purchase of a bottle of water with the unnecessary purchase of a chocolate-flavored PowerBar.

My biggest challenge was one exit away: the seven-mile stretch along Highway 156 West, a secondary road connecting 101 to the Pacific Coast Highway just about ten miles north of Monterey. Having stopped once to quench my thirst and again to satisfy my hunger, I had no more cards to play. A *third* pit stop would sound ridiculous. I took the ramp and merged onto 156, making a reluctant commitment to venture forth into the great unknown.

The two-lane road was straight and narrow. To our left, toward Salinas, wide-open farmland rolled on for miles. To our right, the tall trees and thick foliage lining the highway would have provided the perfect cover for an emergency ditch, but with no shoulder to pull onto, it didn't do me much good.

I reached over and held Cynthia's hand, stared into her spectacular blue eyes, and lied through my teeth. "I know I was a little grouchy when we left, but I really am happy that we're going to Carmel. Thank you for planning everything." If I said it out loud, maybe I'd start to believe it myself.

My words brought a smile to Cynthia's face, but they didn't do a thing for me.

I spent the next several miles in abject terror, watching the odometer, counting down the remaining distance in tenth-of-a-mile increments. I even tried to distract myself by conjuring events even more catastrophic than losing control of my bowels. *What if an oncoming car drifts into our lane and strikes us head-on at seventy miles per hour?* I tried to feel the sensation of being trapped in Cynthia's crushed Taurus, my bones shattered and my flesh on fire. But as grotesque as these ginned-up distractions were, they couldn't push my thoughts of soiling myself out of my head.

Only when we were safely on the Pacific Coast Highway—now at least I could pull over and run into the ocean if need be—did my tension begin to ease and my insides revert to a more relaxed state.

For the first time since we'd left San Francisco, I took in the view, staring wide-eyed at the majestic beauty of the Monterey Peninsula in much the same way, I imagined, Columbus had first gazed upon the New World.

Now, with the difficult journey behind me, I was ready to make sure our first night in Carmel turned out to be as romantic and unforgettable as Cynthia had hoped. Like all the great explorers before me, I was ready to plant my flag.

◆　　　◆　　　◆

Although the dam proved to be far less effective than I'd hoped, I managed to survive the rest of the weekend, including the drive home, without any catastrophic episodes.

With a business trip to Houston coming up, and no better ideas for getting my problem under control, I stayed the course with Pepto. It wasn't perfect, but it was much better than nothing.

Each subsequent trip to Walgreens and Aisle Four was like a scene from the movie *Groundhog Day*, always going down the same way. Choosing to do my shopping during the less-crowded, off-peak hours, I would enter just after 11:00 PM. The store employed many dealers (Walgreens prefers to call them cashiers), but each Pepto purchase matched me with the same one. Her nametag identified her as Vivian.

"Hi. How are you?" was her standard opening line.

This was my cue to direct her attention to my sole purchase, the large, pink bottle sitting on the counter, and shoot her a look designed to say, in no uncertain terms, "How do you *think* I'm doing, Vivian?"

At this point in the scene, the script called for her to deliver a facial expression conveying sudden recognition, followed by a condescending half smile that said, "Oh, right. You're that poor bastard who's bought eight large bottles of Pepto-Bismol in two weeks. Sucks to be you, huh?"

I didn't care for her mocking attitude, but she knew she had the upper hand in this business relationship. We both knew I needed what she had. She knew I'd be back. Following an awkward good-bye, the camera zoomed in for a close-up of the slip of paper Vivian had placed in my hand: "Please visit again."

As I walked onto Divisadero Street, my final line was to myself: "I can't promise you anything, Vivian."

Not only were Vivian and I seeing too much of each other, but she was way too judgmental—a bad trait, in my opinion, for a drug dealer. Luckily she wasn't the only game in town, and I began to take my business elsewhere. Some nights I stopped in at Safeway for my fix. Other nights found me dropping into the minimart sections of the gas stations lining Lombard Street. The family-owned neighborhood corner markets were almost always well stocked with Pepto. My needs were being met. No pressure. No judgment.

Back at home, I had to be careful not to get sloppy. In addition to a kitchen and a wall between our bedrooms, my roommate, Randy, and I also shared a trash can. Frequent sightings of empty Pepto-Bismol bottles, week after week, would be just the kind of evidence that might lead him to think I'd developed an addiction.

In all likelihood, he was already aware that my digestive system operated at a suboptimal level. After all, we also shared a bathroom. But there was no way Randy could have grasped the scope of my issues. The last thing I needed after a hard day at the office was to come home and walk into some type of intervention. "Tim, we're here tonight because we care about you ... and we think you have a problem."

So, like an alcoholic concealing vodka bottles, I went to elaborate measures to dispose of my empties, making frequent use of public garbage cans and the downstairs karaoke bar's recycle buckets. *I don't have a problem. I can stop anytime. I swear.*

The night before leaving for Houston, three things concerned me: my tongue appeared to be permanently stained an unnatural shade of pink; my recreational Pepto use had developed into an expensive daily habit; and the protection offered by the dam was helpful, but never impenetrable.

◆   ◆   ◆

"Hey, are you OK in there?"

"Uh … huh, I'll be right out," I said through the door. I had been holed up in the men's room for a good thirty minutes. Every time I tried to leave, my insides forced me to stay put. No end in sight.

"Great," Jonathan said, "because they're closing up, and we gotta get out of here."

It had seemed like a good idea at the time. Jonathan was a competing mutual fund wholesaler whom I'd met at that conference in Denver. He lived in Houston and was nice enough to show me the nightlife during my first visit to his city. A flashy guy who was always looking to impress the ladies, Jonathan had picked me up at my hotel in his red Porsche. "I hope you like Mexican food."

In truth, I loved the cuisine I had come to know as Mexican food, not yet appreciating the gap in severity between an enchilada eaten in New York or San Francisco and one eaten closer to the border in Houston.

"Chuy's is a lot of fun," he said, "and it's *the* place for people watching, if you know what I mean."

I did.

I wasn't ready to leave the men's room, but I had no choice. I finally opened the door. The beautiful people had left. The party was over. As for people watching, the only people left were the staff, and the only person they were watching was me. I knew what they were thinking: "Why have you been in there so long? And now that you're out, will you please leave so we can go home?"

I must not have been the first out-of-town *gringo* Jonathan had taken to Chuy's. I got the sense that he'd seen it all before. "I should have warned you. The Mexican food down here's got a little bit of a kick to it, if you know what I mean."

Again, I did.

The restaurant's front door slammed shut and was locked behind us. The message was not subtle: "*Adios, gringo.* Good riddance." The toilet at Chuy's was no longer an option. My stomach was still in knots, and another bathroom visit felt inevitable. With great trepidation, I opened the car door and, as if handling a bottle of nitroglycerin, eased my rear end onto the cream-colored, leather seat of my host's brand-new Porsche. Talk about anxiety.

"Hey, partner, why don't we get you back to your hotel? You don't look so hot."

"Yeah, sounds great," I said, "but I'm not sure I can make it that long ... if you know what I mean."

It was hard to say whether he was more concerned about my well-being or his car's interior. Whatever his motive, Jonathan yanked hard on the steering wheel and accelerated this machine into a ninety-degree right turn. I think we pulled four Gs before screeching to a halt. When I opened my eyes, we were parked in front of a Circle K convenience store.

"Hang in there, hoss. I'll be right back. The cavalry is on the way."

In a flash, Jonathan had returned. "This stuff will fix you right up," he said, tossing a brown paper bag into my lap. The package inside was familiar.

"Imodium?" I asked. "Didn't they have any Pepto?"

"Nah, Pepto is kids' stuff. If you're hurtin' as bad as I think you are, *this* is what you want. Everybody uses it. Trust me." He sounded so confident.

Our exchange reminded me of high-school peer pressure. *Don't get me wrong, beer is cool ... but you're gonna* love *how vodka makes you feel. Trust me.*

Hell, if he was willing to risk the alteration of his passenger seat's color scheme, he must have known what he was talking about. *Nothing wrong with a little experimentation, right?* I ripped open the package and swallowed two tablets. We decided to hang around in the parking lot until the pills kicked in.

Shortly after I took my medicine, a precautionary trip to Circle K's toilet confirmed a quick end to my flooding. *This is amazing!* The new stuff built one hell of a dam—and quickly, too. *Can this be legal?*

When Jonathan dropped me off at my hotel, he shook my hand and tossed me the Imodium box. "These are for you, hoss."

"How much do I owe you?" I asked, reaching for my wallet.

"Don't sweat it. This round's on me," he said. "My treat, OK?"

"Thanks, man. I owe you."

I knew Jonathan was right. Pepto *was* kids' stuff, and it just wasn't doing it for me anymore. Now that I'd been turned on to Imodium, there was no going back.

Back in my hotel room, I pulled the tablets out of the box and popped two more into my mouth, just for good measure. I still had a couple of sales calls the next morning, and I needed all the help I could get.

I didn't plan on using Imodium forever, just until I could get things under control … or until I found something stronger.

Empty Promises

I couldn't believe my eyes. As I flipped through the channels, all four local newscasts reported the story. I watched on Channel 4.

ANCHOR: The California Highway Patrol responded to a bizarre incident this morning involving a passenger on an airport shuttle. Our own Steve Henderson has the story. Steve, what can you tell us?

REPORTER: Jessica, at approximately ten o'clock this morning, a Super Shuttle van en route to San Francisco International Airport made an unscheduled stop along Highway 101 South. Eyewitnesses described what happened as passenger revolt.

ANCHOR: I'm sorry, Steve, but are you saying the *passengers* revolted or the passengers *were* revolted?

REPORTER: Jessica, I guess you could say both. Let me explain. It was while the van was stuck in heavy traffic that a male passenger lost complete control—of his bowels. By all accounts, the odor was so horrific that the other five passengers forced him from the vehicle and left him on the side of the highway.

ANCHOR:	Steve, what about the van's driver? Did he just sit and watch this happen?
REPORTER:	Not at all. He held open the doors.
ANCHOR:	What became of that stinky passenger?
REPORTER:	Jessica, CHP is still trying to locate the man they're calling the Olfactory Offender after he fled the scene in shame. We believe his name is Tim Phelan of San Francisco. He is thirty years old, five feet nine, light brown hair, and was last seen wearing heavily stained khaki pants."

Nobody else in San Francisco watched this newscast because it never aired on TV. In my mind, however, it was broadcast more frequently than *It's a Wonderful Life* between Thanksgiving and New Year's.

To avoid such a nightmare from becoming a reality, I chose to drive my own car to SFO instead of opting for any form of shared transportation.

The heavy, bumper-to-bumper traffic I'd experienced on my previous trips to the airport was no fluke. In 1996, the height of the dot-com boom, commuting via the Bay Area's freeways had become a daily exercise in frustration. According to Yahoo, the 15.8-mile ride from my apartment to SFO should take twenty-six minutes—ironic, since hundreds of Yahoo employees spent well over an hour driving along this same congested route each morning. It wasn't a commute—it was a slog.

When you're trapped motionless behind a sea of red brake lights, getting off the freeway to find the nearest restroom is no easy feat. Even driving solo, every airport trip held the requisite elements of a catastrophe in the making.

Back at the office, forces conspired to make my life even more difficult. After I submitted my sixth consecutive expense report that included a receipt for long-term airport parking, it was becoming clear that my employer and I had conflicting agendas.

My objective was to spare no expense in minimizing my anxiety of soiling my boxers en route to SFO. The folks who approved my expense reports, by contrast, were intent on me using the less expensive option of taking Super Shuttle, which only exacerbated my anxiety by giving control of the vehicle to someone else and providing me an audience of strangers. It was a zero-sum game. If I kept driving myself to the airport, their bottom line would suffer. If I gave in and called Super Shuttle, mine would be devastated.

My next business trip, however, marked a turning point. That morning I welcomed the challenges awaiting me on 101 South. For the first time, I would leave my VW parked at home and entrust my safe passage to Super Shuttle. I wasn't coerced by the accounting people. Nor was my decision born out of a newfound concern for my employer's profitability, but rather, I had recently stumbled upon a discovery that promised to make my bowel-related anxieties a thing of the past. I had a new attitude: bring it on!

Hours before the blue and yellow van arrived at my apartment, I was filled with hope. Moments later I would be filled with something else.

Weeks earlier, at the starting line of a local running race, I had vented to my friend Matt about my bowels' resemblance to the never-quite-empty tube of toothpaste.

"Dude, how many trips are you going to make?" Matt was referring to my third visit to the Porta Potty in fifteen minutes.

"I know, it's messed up," I said. "But I can't seem to completely empty my tank before a race." I saw no need to let him know that my digestive issues extended far, far beyond running races.

"Yeah, I hear you," Matt said. "I hate being constipated—*especially* before a race."

Constipated? Matt had always paid selective attention. In this case, the word *completely* had somehow slipped through the conversational cracks. As I was writing off our exchange, he surprised me by offering up a value-added gem.

"Sometimes, if it's really bad," Matt said nonchalantly, "I'll just give myself an enema."

"A *what?*" I was stunned. I knew the term, but I'd always thought of an enema as an antiquated treatment from medicine's dark ages, administered in hospitals to protesting patients by crabby old Nurse Ratched types. What did he mean "give myself an enema?" How? Where? Why?

"An enema. It's easy," he said. "It comes in a little plastic bottle. Squeeze it into your butt and, next thing you know, no more constipation. You are empty and ready to race."

And, I imagined, ready to date, travel, or even ride in a Super Shuttle van.

An enema … brilliant! It seemed so logical, so obvious. Building a dam had been a foolish undertaking. To my great horror, I'd learned the hard way that even a dam built from Imodium was no match for my determined bowels. Not even the strongest Kevlar bulletproof vest could stop the armor-piercing rounds my body produced.

The solution to my problem didn't lie in trying to hold back nature's powerful forces, but rather in assisting and accelerating its powerful flow. I now had the answer: drain the pond. Nothing could possibly flow from my bowels if they were empty. Why hadn't I thought of this? There would be no more toothpaste left. Not in this tube, anyway.

I feared the answer to my next question, but asked anyway. "Where do you buy them?"

◆   ◆   ◆

I was nervous to walk back into Walgreens. I hadn't been there in months, having chosen instead to replenish my stockpiles of Imodium while traveling to different cities in different time zones. I didn't know if she had moved to another store, found another profession, or had pissed off the wrong customer, but I was relieved that Vivian was nowhere to be seen. She would have had a field day with this purchase.

Where did they hide the enemas? I had a hunch, but searched all the pharmacy's other aisles before discovering them in good old Aisle Four. Buying an enema took the concept of embarrassing purchases to a whole new level. It suggested not an upset stomach or heartburn or even diarrhea, but a mysterious ailment even more bizarre. "What in God's name are you going to do with *that* ... you freak?"

As if to satisfy the curiosity of anybody incapable of answering the previous question, the manufacturer had the good sense to adorn the outside of the package with a set of not-so-subtle visual clues.

Below the heading "Positions for using this enema" appeared two figure drawings. The first, entitled "Left-side position," could easily be confused with the police chalk outline drawn around a pedestrian who came to his final rest facedown after being struck by a speeding truck.

The second and more attention-getting diagram, the "Knee-chest position," depicted a naked man with his head on the floor and his raised butt pointing toward the ceiling. Take away the wording, which was small enough to be dwarfed by the drawings, and nine out of ten people would fill in the only logical alternative title: "Man prepares to receive anal sex."

For a few seconds, I entertained the notion of asking the ever-present homeless man camped outside the store to buy the enema for me, like an underage kid asking an adult to buy him liquor. *Hey, mister, can you do me a favor?*

Without resorting to shoplifting, it would be impossible to conceal the enema from view. With my luck, I'd get caught, and I couldn't bear the thought of being written up in the police blotter for stealing an enema. Serving time behind bars would give me plenty of time to perfect the knee-chest position.

Camouflage seemed a wiser and safer option. To disguise my true mission, I filled a shopping basket with unneeded decoys: paper towels, shaving cream, memo pads, and—to put an exclamation point on my heterosexuality—a copy of *Maxim*. *Please don't let me run into anyone I know.* Fortunately the only friends I ran into were Imodium and Pepto-Bismol … but we didn't hang out much anymore.

Having endured yet another self-conscious trip down the aisle, I was eager to get started. It was 8:00 AM—just one hour before my pickup. Even though the process seemed intuitive, I wasn't going to take any chances. I looked at the enema box and read the printed instructions with the same exacting attention that a jittery first-time flier might devote to reading the emergency safety card before takeoff. *Better safe than sorry.* I started reading.

"Uses: For relief of occasional constipation or bowel cleansing before rectal examinations." OK, so I wasn't the ideal target customer for this product. Maybe spending an hour stuck in traffic, trapped with total strangers, might not technically be considered a rectal examination, but it was one of the biggest tests my rectum would ever face—and cleansing my bowels beforehand was the only chance I had to avoid getting a big, fat F.

I revisited my "positions for using this enema" choices. Homo-erotic overtones notwithstanding, I opted for the knee-chest position because it would let gravity guide the enema's 4.5 fluid ounces of saline along a steep, downhill path to the depths of my colon.

With my boxers around my ankles, I was in position, and I jumped ahead to read "How to use this enema." After removing the orange protective cap, I was then supposed to maneuver the lubricated tip, which had the approximate diameter of a number-two pencil, gently into position with a "slight side-to-side movement" that would relax the anus muscles.

The next section puzzled me. It said, "Insertion may be easier if person receiving enema bears down, as if having a bowel movement.

This helps relax the muscles around the anus." The person *receiving* the enema? Did this imply that a second person ought to be in the room *giving* the enema? Matt hadn't mentioned anything about this being a team effort.

I hoped I could pull this off alone because my only option for a helper was my roommate, who hadn't yet left for work. *Hey, Randy, you got a minute?* I wouldn't have to worry about him organizing an intervention. This was the kind of request that led to evictions, even in San Francisco.

Oh, and as for the claim that using the side-to-side movement would relax the muscles around the anus ... well, don't believe everything you read.

Once the tip had been inserted, I squeezed the bottle. According to the directions, "It is not necessary to empty the bottle completely, as it contains more liquid than needed." I forced every last drop out of the bottle.

The next step called for me to remain in the man-prepares-to-receive-anal-sex position until, in the clinical language of the directions, my "need to evacuate" became "strong" (usually two to five minutes). The directions ended there. Presumably I would know what to do from that point on.

Two minutes passed. I felt no change. *Did I miss a step?*

Three minutes. Status quo. *Do enemas have expiration dates?*

Four minutes. It was beginning to work. *I think I feel something. Keep it going.*

Five minutes. My need to evacuate was accelerating. *Cool, but please don't let Randy walk in.*

Six minutes and twenty seconds. *Probably not the time to get hung up on semantics, but how exactly do they define "strong"?*

I looked down at my bedroom's off-white carpeting and made a financial decision. If I was going to have any chance of ever seeing my security deposit again, I couldn't afford to make it any *more* off-white.

It felt like a combination of two horrible sensations: the familiar urgency of uncontrollable diarrhea and the doubled-over pain of getting kicked in the groin. Because nature never intended one body to experience both forms of pain at the same time (not even a sadist would kick a man in the balls when he had explosive diarrhea, would he?), it was a bit overwhelming to process what was happening to my body. Luckily my brain sorted through the sensory fog just in time to remind me of the task at hand.

With both thumbs gripping the inside of my boxers' elastic waistband, I barreled down the narrow hallway to the bathroom. As a first-timer, I hoped my time and distance calculations were accurate.

I couldn't have timed it any better. With no need for effort or straining, the thirty-second process was as involuntary as it was violent, leaving me emptier than a burning movie theater. For perhaps the first time since college, my insides felt hollow. A two-pack of enemas had cost me $1.50. But I would have been happy to pay $1,000.

At long last, I had found a defense that my bowels could not overcome. In a successful preemptive strike, I had drained the pond. Nothing could possibly go wrong. I was bulletproof.

◆   ◆   ◆

The doorbell rang. I was the first of three passengers to be picked up. Having just discovered my silver bullet, I was fearless.

I giddily hopped into the van and assumed the unfamiliar role of worry-free passenger. As the driver and I made our way from my apartment to nearby Pacific Heights to pick up our second passenger, I wasn't just beaming; I felt downright cocky. *Bulletproof. Bring ... it ... on!*

Caught behind a tourist-packed cable car, our van crawled up the steep incline of Hyde Street toward our next stop. When the trolley stopped in front of us at the top of Lombard Street to unload its passengers, we pulled into the driveway of a beautiful apartment building high atop affluent Russian Hill to pick up ours.

After ringing the doorbell, our driver walked back to the van. "The gentleman is running a couple of minutes late. He said it would be a few minutes before he's ready," the driver said.

I took this to mean we were going to wait for him. Not even this unwelcome news, which would only lengthen our trip to the airport, could bother me. *Not today, baby.*

There were worse places to be kept waiting. From my seat, I took in the picturesque panorama—or tried to, at least. My view of San Francisco Bay was obstructed not by the fog, but by the swarm of camera-toting out-of-towners who converged at this spot en masse every day of the year to snap photos of Alcatraz and Coit Tower. As usual, they awaited their turn to descend Lombard Street, aka America's most crooked street, which frequently doubled as America's most crowded street as well. Arriving by rental car, cable car, or (on very rare occasions) on foot, hundreds of vacationers packed the Russian Hill sidewalks and streets as effectively as any of the city's antiwar protests or Gay Pride parades. They were everywhere.

A momentary break in the crowd gave me a bird's-eye view of Alcatraz and a chance to reflect on my recent tour of the former federal penitentiary. It had been Cynthia's idea. She'd been there before, but she'd been adamant that I see "The Rock" for myself.

To Cynthia it was a matter of principle: "You *cannot* live in San Francisco without going to Alcatraz at least once. You just *can't.*"

"Come on, give me a break," I'd said. "That's for tourists, not locals."

But Cynthia would have no part of my transparent appeal to elitism. She was resolute. "We're going."

That wasn't exactly the reward I had expected from her. After Carmel, which had turned out to be the catalyst that took our relationship from "you're really cool to hang out with" to "I love you," I'd opened up and explained—to the best of my ability, anyway—the perplexingly intertwined physical and psychological demons I'd been fighting. I had no idea how she would react. But even though I feared losing her, I felt too close to her to hide such a big secret.

To my great relief, not only did Cynthia not leave me, but she also had a plan to fix me. In concept, her plan was simple.

"You need to face your fears," she'd said. "The sooner you do that, the sooner you'll be back to normal. It's psychological. Trust me … it's all in your head."

And why shouldn't I have trusted her? She was virtually an expert in the field, having taken all of two introductory-level psychology courses in college. In addition to being my girlfriend, Cynthia had now appointed herself my therapist, looking for any and every opportunity to put me in the uncomfortable position of staring down the kinds of situations that scared the crap out me.

Her zeal to cure me was relentless. Taking the ferry to Alcatraz was one of many sessions to which I reluctantly consented. (For the record, the ferry was equipped with plenty of toilets, whereas Alcatraz itself was somewhat less accommodating: even though each of the hundreds of prison cells has its own dedicated toilet, for some reason they're off-limits for tourists.) Earlier ventures included driving headlong into the crowds at Union Square for a day of clothes shopping, crossing the Golden Gate Bridge to eat dinner in Sausalito, and playing golf with her father when he came to town.

Though our forays were somewhat helpful to my confidence after the fact, I wasn't all that crazy about facing my fears; it was hard, nerve-wracking work. An enema, on the other hand, appeared to provide far more benefit with much less unpleasantness. I decided not to tell Cynthia about my enema experiment. I didn't think she'd approve of my abandoning her systematic approach for a quick fix.

After no more than a minute of waiting for our tardy traveler, I knew something was wrong … something more, that was, than the disturbing preponderance of middle-aged couples dressed in matching his-and-hers nylon running suits.

The familiar alarm bells started going off. It was the same sensation that had sent me scurrying to my toilet an hour earlier, but only slightly less intense. I was confused. *I did achieve complete elimination from the enema, didn't I?* Well, apparently not *complete* elimination. This development was unfathomable. How could anything be left?

My newfound feeling of absolute invincibility was short lived. I was scared to death. My palms sweat and my body shook. Panic was setting in. My morning had all the elements of my most dreaded nightmare: an urgent need to go; imprisonment in a Super Shuttle van; broad daylight; concrete city streets teeming with tourists; no public restroom; and the certainty of heavy, stop-and-go traffic. I was having a meltdown, and my need to evacuate—my rectum and the van—was, by any definition, "strong."

"Excuse me, sir?" I said to the driver. "I'm so sorry, but I'm not feeling so hot."

He looked confused. He didn't seem like the type who would fall for my mimed heartburn routine. I held one hand over my stomach and the other over my mouth. "I'm a little nauseous. I need to get some air. I'll be right back."

It was the best explanation I could come up with on short notice. What was my plan? I had no idea. I figured I had at least a couple of minutes to work with before our fashionably late friend emerged from his luxury apartment and graced us with his presence. All I knew was that whatever I was going to do, it would best be done somewhere else. I sprinted from the van, taking no notice of the reactions of the driver or the other passenger.

In stark contrast to the tourists creeping down the steep twists and turns of America's most crooked street at a close-to-constipated pace, my fecal matter was performing its best impression of a world-record-seeking Olympic bobsled team, negotiating my colon's slick S-turns and switch-backs with reckless abandon at breakneck speed. With no public restroom in sight, it appeared I was going to lose this race against the clock—in dramatic fashion. *The agony of defeat!*

On this inhospitable mountaintop of concrete, my salvation appeared before me. Although I had never noticed it before, catty-corner from the top of the crooked street was a small public park.

The park wasn't even really a park, but rather one tennis court that was surrounded at its perimeter by not nearly enough trees. I bolted toward the most promising thicket and made the best of a horrible situation. Even with so many tourists milling about, I still thought I had a good chance of concealing my activity.

I saw him about five seconds before he saw me. He was a short, elderly man with one eye closed and the other squinting through his camcorder's viewfinder, panning his camera in a counterclockwise sweep from the Presidio to Pacific Heights.

We were on a clear collision course, but I had neither the time nor the will to take any sort of evasive action. Staring into the camera, he would remain oblivious to my presence until it was too late. I was a good fifty feet away, but his zoom lens could make it look like three. I lowered my head to hide my face but managed to sneak a sideways glance through my fingers to watch his reaction.

I'll never know why, but after his entire body flinched, the man continued to point the camera in my direction for three or four more seconds. I guess I didn't care what he did with the footage—as long as he didn't turn it over to any of the TV news stations.

As he walked away, I completed my mission, dumbfounded by how far my body had been from being empty. It was like opening the door to a one-car garage and watching two enormous eighteen-wheel trucks drive out. It didn't make any sense.

My Boy Scout training from so many years ago was now paying off. I was able to rip an ample number of leaves from the closest tree and complete my cleanup.

Since my second urge had come out of nowhere, I pondered the likelihood of a third. If I had learned anything, it was that feeling empty was different than being empty. I no longer had any idea what to expect from my body, but I did have a flight to catch.

"Are you feeling better?" asked our driver.

"Yeah, much better, thanks."

I climbed back into the van, limbs still shaking, and prayed today would not mark my TV news debut. I turned to my fellow passengers. "Sorry for holding everyone up. Thanks for waiting." It was as much of a sincere apology as it was an attempt to have them think of me as a nice person. If they liked me, then even if I did suffer an out-of-body experience before we arrived at SFO, maybe they wouldn't be as quick to throw me from the van.

What I hoped would be a permanent solution proved a major set-back, causing far more harm than good. Spending the remainder of the forty-five-minute drive waiting for the third turd to drop, I berated myself for not anticipating this disastrous turn of events. While I had certainly expected the enema to set off a major quake, I just hadn't been prepared for the devastating aftershocks.

Far from being yesterday's news, in my mind's eye the story of the Olfactory Offender would remain an ongoing headline.

Driving a Hard Bargain

It started out as a simple, loving gesture.

"Do you want a ride to the airport on Monday?" Cynthia asked.

"I'd love one," I told her. "Are you heading down that way for a meeting?"

"No, but since you're going to be gone all week, I thought it would be nice to spend a little more time together and then see you off with a kiss."

Lucky for me, Cynthia worked from her apartment and was free to arrange her schedule as she wished.

In just under two years, our relationship had come a long way. Not only had I lost my fear of driving with Cynthia, even in heavy traffic, but I had also come to regard her as my personal security blanket. I had never come out and told her, but nobody else made me feel as comfortable and accepted as she did.

Her offer couldn't have come at a better time. Because my company would no longer pay for airport parking, and I vowed never again to set foot in another Super Shuttle van as long as I lived, I had to find a new way to get to SFO. The company was willing to cover the cost of a cab ride, but that wasn't much help. With only me and the driver in the taxi, the source of any foul odors would be obvious. It was safe to say that if your cab smelled like an unflushed toilet, business might fall off a bit—just the kind of concern that might lead a cab driver to violence.

The night before my trip, Cynthia invited me over to her place for a home-cooked meal. Several months earlier, she had begun to supplement her aggressive face-your-fears campaign with a new treatment approach that focused on my unhealthy diet.

According to her hypothesis, my digestive tract was more likely to behave normally if I replaced my steady intake of pizza, burgers, and other greasy, fried foods with fish, chicken, and maybe an occasional fruit or vegetable. Despite my protests that I'd never once noticed a link between my attacks and eating any particular food (I categorized coffee as a beverage, not food), I went along with it anyway. But so far, other than producing a sharp increase in intestinal gas, eating healthier was no more effective at taming my insides than anything else I'd tried.

Falling asleep the night before a flight was always a challenge, my insomnia guaranteed by the usual suspects: the airport check-in line, the security line, the backed-up jetway, the tarmac traffic … and of course the evil seat belt sign. But this time, it was nice not to have to worry about the drive to the airport.

At week's end, when I walked out of baggage claim and onto the curb, Cynthia stood waiting. She hurried toward me with her wide smile and open arms.

I gave her a big hug, holding her tightly. "It's good to be back."

"I missed you," she said.

"I missed you, too," I told her, meaning every word of it.

I walked back and threw my bags into the trunk of her waiting Taurus. Walking toward the passenger-side door, I watched scores of returning travelers march out of baggage claim and hop into the yellow taxis and Super Shuttle vans that filled the curbside loading zone.

They looked so calm, so nonchalant about the journeys they were about to undertake. If they had any worries, surely they were of the mundane variety, nuisance-type stuff: *Will I make it to Whole Foods before it closes? Should I upgrade to a bigger SUV? How am I going to pay for my kids to go to college?* Did they even know, I wondered, how good they had it? Probably not.

As I got into the car, what Cynthia had intended to be a one-time, or maybe occasional, luxury had now become a necessity for me. I would have to find a way to make this biweekly chauffeur service permanent. There was simply no other way.

I leaned across the seat and gave her a kiss. "I don't know what I did to deserve it, but thank you so much for picking me *and* dropping me off. How about Pomodoro tonight?"

Even though it wasn't fancy or expensive, Pasta Pomodoro, the one on Union Street, was Cynthia's favorite restaurant. That was one of the traits I loved most about her: she was down-to-earth and practical, a rarity in trendy, fashion-conscious San Francisco. After what she'd done for me, treating her to a special meal was the least I could do to show my appreciation. And if my inexpensive but thoughtful expression of gratitude just happened to increase the likelihood of more airport rides … well then, so much the better.

I pulled out all the stops. "We can have a bottle of cabernet … that shrimp fettuccine you like so much … and maybe some tiramisu."

She broke into another huge smile. "Mmmmm, that sounds perfect."

Two weeks later, I was headed off once again, this time to North Carolina. Hoping that I would encounter less runway congestion and more empty seats on the plane, I had begun to schedule myself on late-morning flights, well after the airport's hectic morning rush hour. With a little luck, maybe I could even get my very own row back by the lavatory.

"Honey," I asked, "what does your schedule look like next Tuesday?"

"Pretty busy," she said. "Why?"

I said, "Oh, I was wondering if you would be able to do me a huge favor."

She looked suspicious. "*How* huge?"

"Well," I said with a sheepish grin, "could you give me a ride to the airport?"

"I just gave you a ride last week," she said. "You want me to take you *again?*"

"Please?" I asked, piling on the sweet, boyish charm.

Cynthia thumbed through her Day-Timer. "I'll have to reschedule a conference call and a meeting. So I guess I *could* …"

"*Please?*" Now I was narrowing the gap between playful neediness and begging. "We can go to Pomodoro again."

"You better appreciate me," she said with a steely gaze.

"I do. I promise," I assured her.

As the weeks passed, my request for a *third* ride met stiff resistance. Even the promise of Pomodoro had lost its persuasive punch.

She asked the obvious question. "Why don't you take a cab?"

"I can't do that," I said.

"But you said you can expense it." She was starting to lose her patience. "You'd rather have me blow off my work and give you a ride instead of taking a cab that your company is willing to *pay* for?"

I still hadn't told her about the Super Shuttle disaster or my ill-fated foray into enemas. Nor had I shared the fact that cab rides were every bit as capable of triggering the sudden onset of my symptoms as our first trip to Carmel. Now I had no choice but to pull back the curtain of vulnerability a bit more. Even if this wrinkle wouldn't come as a surprise to her, it would still be new information.

It was strange. I'd devoted the previous nine years of my life to analyzing every last detail of my bathroom fears and theorizing on all conceivable causes and cures. Hell, I thought about this stuff more than sex. And yet the right words were now difficult to find and even tougher to articulate.

Why is it so important for Cynthia to drive me to the airport? Why did I refuse to take a cab? Such simple questions. I could hear fragments of explanations buzzing wildly around my head like too many flies circling last week's trash. I reached out and grabbed the first one I was lucky enough to snare.

"I'm comfortable around you," I said, realizing this wasn't a good answer to her question.

Cynthia didn't say anything. She looked puzzled.

I explained that as long as I was with her—and *only* her—it didn't matter if we were stuck in traffic. My backside was cool. I confessed that cab rides terrified me because I couldn't count on strangers to be as understanding to me as she was.

"You make me feel safe because you accept me for who I am … bathroom issues and all," I said. "Nobody else, not even my family, makes me feel that way. Do you understand what I'm saying?"

Maybe it struck a chord in her inner nurturer, or maybe she (correctly) interpreted my confession as a breakthrough to a higher level of intimacy between us.

As her blue eyes welled up, Cynthia nodded as she swallowed the lump in her throat. "Yes," she said with her voice cracking. "I do."

Effective immediately, my private-car service was reinstated in perpetuity.

◆   ◆   ◆

Lest I give you the impression our relationship was lopsided, I should point out I wasn't the only one driven by a need that some might consider irrational. As badly as I wanted rides to the airport, Cynthia wanted to be not just a bride, but a *young* bride.

Maybe she'd been talking this way since the day we met, but I had only recently begun to pick up on it. With increasing frequency, I began hearing the phrase "meeting and marrying." Cynthia would say things like, "My sister *met and married* her husband within nine months," or "It only took one year for my brother and his wife to *meet and marry.*"

She never came out and said what her exact expectations were as far as we were concerned, but the implication was clear: the shorter the total elapsed time between telling somebody, "Hello, how do you do?" and vowing before God and family to spend the rest of your life together with a promise of "I do," the better your chances for a happy marriage.

I had no qualms about getting married. But because I wanted to make sure Cynthia was the right person and we were together for the right reasons, I was in no great rush. A good friend of mine had recently advised me to take my time, adding, "Remember, your spouse is the only family member you get to choose." But buying much more time would not be easy. After dating her for two years, I got the feeling that Cynthia was on the verge of stamping our relationship with an expiration date.

◆　　　◆　　　◆

As we drove through the Presidio, a heavy afternoon fog poured into the bay, closing the curtain on what had been a rare balmy Sunday.

The red light on Cynthia's cell phone was blinking. "It's probably just my boss calling about our meeting tomorrow," she said.

As Cynthia checked her voice mail, I watched in awe as the dark wall of fog engulfed the massive Golden Gate Bridge before our eyes. It happened all the time, but up close it looked even more surreal. It wouldn't be long before we found ourselves enshrouded, too. Along with the rare San Francisco thunderstorm, this was the kind of weather event that always brought out the wide-eyed little girl in Cynthia. I looked over to watch her reaction.

Cynthia gazed down at the floor, too preoccupied with listening to her message to even notice. I watched her expression change from ho-hum to disbelief. *Is something wrong, or is this good news?* I tapped her on the shoulder, pointing out the unfolding natural drama. She spun around, shoved my hand away, and hissed at me like a coiled cobra. In her eyes, I saw shock … and, if I wasn't mistaken, anger. Raw anger. *What could her boss have possibly said?*

Cynthia closed her phone and slammed it back into her purse. Just like that, the shock and anger were replaced by joy and excitement—*obviously forced*, I thought.

"That was Olivia," she said, swallowing hard to keep her true emotions, whatever they were, in check. "She's … engaged. Scott proposed this morning. My roommate's getting married! Can you believe it?"

"No, I sure can't," I said with total sincerity.

But if *I* couldn't believe it, then Cynthia *really* couldn't believe it. Olivia and Scott (who lived and worked in Atlanta) had a bicoastal relationship and had been dating every other weekend for almost four months. Cynthia's best friend for years, Olivia was twenty-eight and had a long history of being relationship-challenged. Not only had she never been in love, she'd never even had a boyfriend.

But now, as Cynthia would see with her own bulging eyes a few hours later, Olivia had a huge rock (tacky, Cynthia would privately point out again and again, but huge nonetheless) on her finger. That Cynthia had been passed by so quickly in her race to the altar and by the most unlikely dark horse of all—she never even considered Olivia a fellow competitor—was more than a tragedy. It was a call to action.

On that foggy afternoon, it was difficult for me to see how Olivia's engagement would impact my life. In time I would look back and realize this development did not *cause* what happened next, only *accelerated* it. Either way, it was the kind of thing I could have lived without.

In the following weeks, I noticed changes in Cynthia's behavior. Gone, for example, were the days of hassle-free airport rides. In fact, she grew increasingly hostile to the idea of rearranging her work schedule to accommodate what she began to refer to as my special needs.

She'd say things like, "It's not really going to be convenient for me to take you next week. Sorry."

And I'd come back with responses like, "How can you say that? You *know* how important this is to me. You *know* I *can't* take a cab."

She had me by the balls, and she knew it. That was when things started getting nasty. "Hey, what happened to facing your fears? How are you ever going overcome them if I keep coddling you?"

"Coddling? What are you saying?" I'd fume.

"What I'm saying is, it would be *nice* if you started to act like a *man*," she'd said once, and implied on several more occasions.

Ouch.

In the end, she would drive me, but the whole thing was puzzling. Why was she raking me over the coals and making me jump through all these hoops? Anytime we got into an argument, she knew exactly how to get her way.

"You've got to be kidding me. We are *not* going to watch *Driving Miss Daisy*," I said as we roamed the aisles at Blockbuster.

"Oh, I think we are …" she said with mocking sweetness, "*if* you still want me to take you to the airport next week."

I had no choice. Like Superman in the face of Kryptonite, I was powerless. To me this was life and death. To Cynthia it was a bargaining chip … and video rentals and pizza toppings were just the beginning. I wondered what would come next. So far she hadn't made that clear. Or if she had, I hadn't heard it.

Olivia had already stunned Cynthia with her overnight mastery of "meeting and marrying." Now, by mailing out her wedding invitations only four weeks after her engagement, she seemed intent on leaving Cynthia in the dust. Like her ring, Olivia's wedding promised to be quite the spectacle: top hats and tails for the groomsmen; horse-drawn carriage for the bride; black tie for the guests.

Judging from her envious reaction, I started to get the sense that Cynthia was more interested in getting married than being married. This was ironic, since my views on the matter were exactly the opposite.

Cynthia and I had attended a handful of weddings together, and at each one, I sat as close to an aisle and the back of the church as possible. While putting my time in captivity to good use by praying for a quick ceremony, I tried to imagine how—if the day ever came—I would ever be able to survive my own wedding.

In all seriousness, being able to endure my time at the altar, in front of my friends and family, and in front of my fiancée's friends and family, without excusing myself to use the toilet was no small hurdle to tying the knot. Brides had certainly been left at the altar before—grooms, too—but surely none had suffered the indignation of being left at the altar for a trip to the bathroom.

If I had reason to suspect Cynthia was obsessed with Olivia's fast-approaching nuptials before, our next trip to the movies confirmed it.

"Can't we see *Air Force One*?" I asked, knowing full well I lacked the necessary leverage.

"Sorry, not tonight," Cynthia said. "I've already made up my mind, and it is not negotiable."

"OK," I said, slinking my way up to the ticket window and pulling out a twenty. "Two adults for *My Best Friend's Wedding,* please." At least the theater wasn't crowded, so I had no trouble securing an aisle seat.

For weeks Cynthia continued to sit back and stew. This was supposed to be *her* time. She was the one who had already invested two years. She had been next in line, not Olivia. Why, Cynthia wondered out loud, was she not married, or at least engaged, yet?

❖   ❖   ❖

A week before Thanksgiving, Cynthia asked me, "How do you feel about us moving in together?"

"Hmmm … I hadn't really given it much thought," I admitted. "Since we've never talked about it before, I didn't know it was something you were interested in."

"I wasn't, but lately I've been giving it more thought. At some point, we're going to have to take the next step, right?" she asked.

I nodded and hoped that answering her second question would let me dodge the first. "Yes, of course."

Cynthia stared into my eyes. "So?"

I played dumb. "So … what?"

"*Are* you willing to think about getting our own place?"

"Yes, of course I'll think about it," I said.

Cynthia looked pleased. "Thank you. That makes me happy."

The way I heard it, Cynthia hadn't issued any kind of ultimatum. No, I was pretty sure she had asked me to do nothing more than *think* about moving in together. And true to my word, I did think about it. In fact, throughout early December, I thought about it a lot.

I could still remember the pain of breaking up with Sarah. When she moved out, it felt like a divorce. I didn't want to go through that again unless I was absolutely sure where things were headed. I concluded if I wasn't ready to marry Cynthia, then I wasn't ready to move in with Cynthia. Not yet, anyway.

A few weeks later, days before we left to spend the holidays with our respective families, Cynthia raised the topic again.

"Have you given it any more thought?" she asked.

"Yes," I said. After explaining how painful my previous experience in this area had been, I said, "I think moving in together is a good idea, but I don't think we should do it just yet."

Cynthia didn't say a word.

"Maybe in a few months," I offered.

"Sure," she said, "but I can't guarantee I'll still be around in a few months."

Now this was stronger than an idle threat, but in my opinion, it still fell short of an ultimatum. I spent the next week with my family in Connecticut and pondered the situation even more.

Why wasn't I ready to marry Cynthia? What was holding me back?

I loved that Cynthia was down-to-earth and adventurous. I loved that she expanded my horizons by pushing me to face my fears. Even though I never appreciated it until after the fact, I loved that she got me to experience things I never would have on my own. I felt like a better person for it.

Even though I hoped I would make more progress under her continued tutelage, I still couldn't envision the day when I'd be able to keep pace with her as an equal. After dietary changes, Imodium, and facing my fears didn't cure whatever was wrong with me, I felt it was inevitable that, despite her gargantuan efforts to prod me forward, I would end up holding her back. This gap, I feared, would always be a source of friction between us.

Still, whether or not Cynthia and I were right for each other, it was depressing to think about being without her. For one thing, if I walked away, I would have to start dating again.

How many anxiety-filled first dates would I have to go on before meeting someone I might click with, and how many more months before I could re-create the comfort level I had with Cynthia? I would be facing a minimum sentence of two to three months of exactly the kind of hell that drove my bowels batty.

I wasn't ready to get married, but clearly I was not ready to let go, either. Right or wrong, I had made my decision: to protect my heart and bowels, I would stay in this relationship as long as I could.

Two weeks later, in early January, Cynthia called and asked me to come over to her apartment.

"Sure, I'll be right over," I said. "What's up?"

"I have something I want to talk about," she said. "I'll tell you when you get here."

When I walked through her door, Cynthia had a distant look on her face. I could tell something was wrong.

"Have a seat," she said.

I did.

"I feel like I've given you every opportunity to move forward and take the next step," she said, "and I've decided I can't wait for you anymore. This is hard for me because I still love you, but it's time for me to move on. I'm sorry."

My barrage of last-minute pleas fell on deaf ears. Not even my desperate promise to put a small-but-tasteful engagement ring on her finger by week's end or my vow to spend the upcoming weekend looking for two-bedroom rentals in Sausalito could sway her. My security blanket had been yanked from my hands, and it was not negotiable.

Not only would I be lonely, heartbroken, and anxious, I would also have to find a new way to get to the airport.

Misery Loves Company

Steve stepped up and took the lead. "Jack and Coke for me, and a vodka tonic for my friend."

I pulled out a twenty and threw it onto the bar. Steve's hand pounced onto the bill and tossed it back as if it were a live grenade. "Sorry. Your money is no good tonight."

The bartender appeared with our cocktails. "Anything else?"

Steve looked at me, raising his eyebrows. I shrugged. "It couldn't hurt." After all, this was a celebration.

"Two shots of Jäger, please."

The fact that I winced at drinking a capful of Pepto-Bismol but savored the cough syrup flavor of Jägermeister proved there was no accounting for taste.

It wasn't easy to find someone to join me for an ice-cold shot of Jäger. I'd always believed people entered your life for a reason. Steve loved Jäger every bit as much as I did. Not surprisingly, a friendship was formed.

Steve made an encapsulated toast. "Here's to your birthday, your new apartment, and your new job. Cheers." We slammed the empty glasses down and motioned for another round. If ever a drink was capable of putting hair on your chest, this was it. *Froufrou* did not apply. This was a man's drink.

The term soul mate is a wholly inappropriate way to describe any platonic connection shared by two heterosexual men, but from early on, it was clear Steve and I had far more in common than loving Jäger, growing up in New York, and working in the investment business.

Our taste in women was similar enough to be at times problematic. In a bar full of single females, we were wingmen who often competed for the same target. Also uncanny was how frequently we arrived at a bar or restaurant wearing the same shirt-and-pants color combo.

We found ways to work through these glitches. It was decided that we would resolve all future women disputes like the men that we were: with a game of rock, paper, scissors (best two out of three, all outcomes binding). To avoid looking like coordinated twins, we began all nights out on the town with a phone call and a decidedly unmasculine question: "What are you wearing?"

After two rounds of shots, Steve excused himself. "I'll be right back … I hope."

As he walked toward the men's room, I was a little buzzed and somewhat confused. What did he mean by *I hope*? We hadn't even begun to drink yet. He couldn't be getting sick. It was only eight o'clock. We still had another four hours to celebrate my thirty-fourth birthday.

He returned a full five minutes later. "Sorry about that."

"Everything go OK in there?" I was as curious as I was concerned. He didn't look as if he had thrown up.

"Yeah. Just having some *issues* tonight," he said. My antenna picked up on something in his tone and body language—something familiar. It was the strained smile and the nervous chuckle when he said *issues*. It sounded exactly like something I would have said. My instincts told me to dig a little deeper.

I picked up my shovel. "*Issues*, huh?"

"I guess you could say I have a very sensitive stomach." Another nervous half smile suggested that this was more than just a case of having a bad day, like with a bout of food poisoning.

With both hands, I thrust the shovel back into the soil. "Has your stomach always been like that?"

Steve shook his head. "No, only over the last couple of years. I didn't really notice it until I moved back to New York, after college."

He sipped on his Jack and Coke, wearing the expression of a lab rat who was all too ready for the evil scientists to cease their prodding and let him out from underneath the microscope. The examination almost died on the spot. But then he added, "At least I wasn't on a plane or in a meeting this time."

"I'm sorry, time-out here," I said. "Planes? Meetings? I'm afraid I'm going to have to ask you to elaborate."

He stared through his drink, and then rolled his eyes skyward, searching for the right words. How much was he willing to reveal, even to a close friend? A long pause preceded his reluctant admission.

He went on to explain how his *issues* always cropped up at the worst times, and with startling urgency. He recounted some of his in-flight emergencies and close calls he'd had during job interviews.

"The scariest part is that it's so unpredictable," Steve said. "It's like everything can be fine for weeks or even months, and then it comes back, out of nowhere. I don't know if it's something I'm eating or what, but it sucks."

Pay dirt!

"Has it ever popped up on a date?" I asked.

Steve's eyes widened as he let out a sigh. "A few weeks ago, I was driving back from Berkeley with that girl ... Gloria. I told you about her, right? Anyway, we were on our way back from dinner. I was doing fine until we hit traffic on the Bay Bridge. I almost exploded in my car."

I couldn't believe what I was hearing. "Really?"

"But the worst time for me is the morning after a girl spends the night. You know how close my bathroom is to my bed. If I used the toilet, she would be able to hear everything. I usually wait until after I drive her home. Believe me, I've had some terrifying drives across town. Have you ever noticed this city isn't exactly packed with public restrooms?"

I nodded. "Uh-huh."

As far as self-affirming moments went, this was second only to that wonderful day in seventh grade when I learned I wasn't the only guy in the world who masturbated. I was still convinced I was a freak, but now at least I wasn't the *only* freak. Were there more of us out there?

"Interesting," was all I could mutter.

Steve sat there, out on a limb, all alone, wondering if his confession had crossed some line, maybe revealed too much. "Sorry, I didn't mean to ramble on about my problems."

It was time to return the favor. "Steve, you're probably not going to believe this, but I've had the exact same problem for years. I can relate to *everything* you just said. Have you ever talked about this with anyone before?"

"No, I can safely say this is a first," Steve said. "You?"

"Before tonight I'd only told one other person," I said.

Now, there's nothing unusual about two guys discussing crass topics like bodily functions at a bar—or anywhere else, for that matter. And on those occasions when men discuss the size, smell, or color of their solid waste, it is typically done in the same boastful way they brag about the size of their penis or the fish they caught. *You should have seen this thing!*

It is much rarer to hear two men swapping confessions about their dysfunction in this department. Not even men who watch *Oprah* or *Dr. Phil* are likely to admit these kinds of inadequacies.

To our mutual amazement, we had found yet another piece of common ground over which we both squatted. For the next half hour, Steve and I sat at the bar and talked at length about the sad state of our stools.

◆   ◆   ◆

The next morning, I woke up to a strange noise. It was a rattling sound. I opened my eyes just in time to see my two lamps, my alarm clock, and my TV wildly vibrating in harmony, doing a little synchronized dance reminiscent of the Electric Slide. *That's strange. When did they learn to do that?* Seconds later, as quickly as it began, the hoedown ended.

Later that morning, I called Steve. "Did you feel it?"

"Feel what?" he asked.

"The earthquake. This morning. Didn't you feel it?" I asked again.

When I had moved to San Francisco, I was well aware of the city's history with earthquakes, and like most newcomers, I lived in constant anticipation of the Big One. But after scurrying to the safety of the nearest door frame for the fiftieth time, only to find out my walls were shaking because the garbage truck was barreling down the block, I stopped worrying about when the unsteady ground beneath my feet might decide to act up and bury me beneath the rubble of a collapsed building. What was the sense of losing sleep over something that happened every ten or twenty years?

"Nope, sure didn't. Was it big?" He didn't sound particularly interested.

"No, not really. It only lasted ten seconds or so. Still kind of cool, though."

People had told me to expect this kind of thing. Now that I had spent my first night in my new apartment, I understood. Steve lived up the hill in Pacific Heights—on the more stable ground known as bedrock. I now lived in the Marina District, a beautiful, posh neighborhood built atop a wobbly foundation of unsteady landfill.

To live in the Marina is to feel *all* of the earth's shudders in magnified fashion—even those that your bedrock-dwelling neighbors never even notice. But it was about more than feeling the ground shift below you; in the 1989 Loma Prieta quake, several homes and apartment buildings on my new block had collapsed into the street and then burned to the ground.

"Still want to go out tonight?" I asked.

"Well, no sense wasting a Saturday night at home. I'll swing by and check out your new pad. See you around eight?"

The chase was still fun, but with each passing week, starting the dating game from scratch was becoming much less enjoyable. Like me, Steve also wanted to get married and start a family. We joked about how neither of us wanted to show up at our children's high-school graduations as eighty-year-old men. Our never-ending quest yielded plenty of dates, but we had yet to meet our future wives.

We usually stayed "on campus"—our term for staying in the neighborhood and hitting the same bars and running into the same people night after night. "Why go farther than we have to?" was usually how I explained my preference to stay local.

As Steve had correctly pointed out, finding a public toilet on a moment's notice was not something you could count on in San Francisco. Straying "off campus" to hang out in the Haight or the Mission (each destination was popular, hip, and fifteen minutes away by cab) meant rolling the dice. I wondered if Steve felt the same way.

Steve showed up, and I gave him the tour.

From the leather chair in my living room, he stared at the unobstructed view of the Golden Gate Bridge two miles to the west. At the end of each day, when it wasn't foggy, the bright orange sun hovered just below the bridge's arching silhouette before plunging into the cold blue of the Pacific.

From the couch, my window provided the perfect frame for the Palace of Fine Arts. The colossal dome sat two blocks away, but it looked as if you could open the window and climb right onto it. At night, all lit up, the landmarks appeared even more dazzling, especially from my rooftop, which boasted a chilly but memorable 360-degree view.

"Nice!" he exclaimed, envious of what was perhaps the ultimate bachelor pad. "How much more are you paying?"

"A little more than double, but it's three times the space. And, I'm not trying to sound like a big shot, but it also comes with a parking spot in the garage downstairs."

Thanks to my new job, I found myself on firm enough financial footing to leave my shoebox of a junior one-bedroom apartment behind. More than a few women, my mother included, had suggested upgrading to a more elegant apartment would be an asset when it came to dating.

"Who cares about the earthquakes and the high rent? This place is incredible. Even if a girl isn't that into you, she'll probably come back just to hang out here."

"Wait, I haven't even shown you the best part," I said.

Whoever designed the floor plan must have shared my strong preference for personal privacy. An absurdly spacious twelve-by-twelve foyer separated the bathroom door from the living room, the dining room, the kitchen, and the bedroom.

I pointed out the obvious: "You're so far away, nobody can hear a thing. It's a built-in embarrassment buffer. How's that for peace of mind?"

"Oh, that reminds me," Steve said. "I came across an article today. It was about a book on IBS."

"IBS? What's that?"

"Irritable bowel syndrome," he said.

"Irritable *brow* syndrome?" I asked, wondering what my thick, unruly eyebrows had to do with anything.

"No, not *brow*. It's *bowel*. Irritable *bowel* syndrome. Apparently it's a medical condition," he said. "I'd never heard of it, either."

I wasn't exactly sure what a *syndrome* was, but I would have been hard pressed to pick two words that more accurately conveyed the nature of my persistent anguish than *irritable* and *bowel*. I was thirty-four years old and, to the best of my knowledge, this was the first time in my life I'd ever heard these three words used in the same sentence.

I didn't want to jump to conclusions, but Steve's inadvertent discovery had Holy Grail written all over it.

I asked, "Do you think that's what we have?"

"I don't know, but it sounds like it's worth checking out."

Indeed.

"Ready to head out and meet our future ex-girlfriends?" I asked.

"Yeah, but can I use your bathroom first?"

"Knock yourself out."

◆   ◆   ◆

My new employer, LPM Investments, prided itself on being a forward-thinking company, and the most glaring expression of this contemporary attitude was the nontraditional look of its workspace. There were no private offices, no cubicles, and no dividers. Every phone call, personal or business, might as well have been an office-wide conference call. Every e-mail, whether sent or received, might as well have been CC'd to the entire floor.

The open architecture suggested—screamed—an egalitarian work-place without walls, figurative or literal, where everybody was, if not exactly equal, then at least equally exposed.

On Monday morning, I got into the office around six o'clock. It was the only way to get any privacy. By seven the place would be teeming with workaholics eager to put in face time and turn every-body else's business into their own.

The right thing to do, of course, was to call Dr. Olson. Yes, I was sure of it. He had gone to med school and studied for years. He was a bona fide expert, armed with the training and knowledge to tell me if I had IBS or not. And if that was his diagnosis ... well then, I would shell out a few bucks for the cure and get back to conquering the world.

But sometimes it's tough to do the right thing, even when you know what it is. The more I thought about it, the less inclined I was to bother my doctor with something that I might not even have. How exactly would I explain my symptoms to him?

It wasn't like I urgently had to go to the bathroom *all* the time—only *some* of the time. And my digestive demons usually attacked only when I knew I couldn't easily get to a bathroom ... or, as had increasingly become the case, when I found myself thinking about such scenarios. The rest of the time, I was relatively issue-free. When I tried to articulate my problem to myself, my physical symp-toms notwithstanding, it sounded more mental than medical. I didn't want Dr. Olson to think I was a hypochondriac or a complete nut job—or both.

So instead I did the next best thing.

Steve didn't remember the name of the book he'd read about. No matter. I fired up my computer and set a course for Amazon.com. I punched in "IBS" and hit Search. Honestly I wasn't expecting to find much information on what I assumed had to be an uncommon disorder.

To my surprise, I didn't find one book on irritable bowel syndrome. I found fifty.

That's right, fifty. As in five zero. It wasn't as if I'd been living in a cave. I watched TV. I read newspapers and magazines. I knew I hadn't exactly asked anybody about the possible existence of such a disorder, but I hadn't asked anybody about colon cancer, bladder infections, yeast infections, or erectile dysfunction, either. Yet I was well aware of them (not firsthand, mind you). This was like not knowing about McDonald's. Why hadn't anybody told me?

Everything I learned about IBS I learned from the online back-cover descriptions of these self-help tomes. I completed my crash course in about forty-five minutes. As I clicked on title after title, each pitch was more or less the same.

"Do you suffer from these symptoms: Diarrhea? Constipation? Diarrhea and constipation? A feeling of urgency? A feeling of incomplete elimination? Abdominal pain or discomfort? Bloating or distension?"

"If so, you may be one of millions ..."

"This book can help by showing you how ..."

I probably didn't have an objective mindset going into this search process. I was an outcast looking to belong. I so badly wanted to think that my symptoms could be explained by a legitimate medical condition that I would have believed anything.

I knew I didn't have *all* the symptoms. Constipation, for example, was a foreign concept to me—something I'd only read about. No, I only had *some* of them. But this was a club I wanted to belong to. One book said ten million Americans had IBS; another claimed the number was closer to fifty-eight million.

If my doctor found that I didn't have IBS, then I'd be right back at square one, on the outside, in freak town.

Browsing through the sea of self-help titles, I got the impression that treating this disorder—much like do-it-yourself home-improvement projects—was something I could ... well ... do myself.

It reminded me of the old ads for the Time-Life books that told millions of TV viewers that paying expensive hourly fees to plumbers, electricians, and carpenters was an outrageous waste of money. By following the easy-to-follow pictures and instructions, you, too, could rewire your home's electrical system or install new plumbing. It was easy.

So too, I was led to believe, was treating IBS.

Somebody once told me a little knowledge was a dangerous thing. In retrospect this would have been the ideal time to heed this cautionary truism. But no—I'd seen all I needed to see, and I knew all I needed to know. I promptly diagnosed myself with irritable bowel syndrome. Then I did what any self-respecting man would do: I set out to fix it.

It wasn't a perfect diagnosis, but where was the danger in a little tinkering? If it didn't work ... well then, it didn't work. I wouldn't be any *worse* off—I read that IBS wasn't fatal. Besides, this time around, my approach would be different. I wouldn't be flying blind. My days of experimenting with outlandishly ill-conceived treatment methods like enemas and Pepto overdoses were over. Thanks to Amazon.com, I now had fifty different roadmaps to help me get my life back on track.

I knew I'd made the mistake of setting my hopes too high in the past, but I had a particularly good feeling about this new strategy. In my mind, the question wasn't if I would conquer my condition, but when.

It wasn't until I started to fill my virtual shopping cart with the most promising self-help titles that I noticed what could prove to be a glitch in my plan.

Eating for IBS was one of a dozen books whose title suggested that dietary changes were the solution.

But I also saw books like *Hypnosis for IBS* and *Irritable Bowel Syndrome and the Mind-Body/Brain-Gut Connection*, whose titles reflected a much different approach.

Seemingly at odds with all of the above were *Curing IBS Naturally with Chinese Medicine* and *The Bible Cure for IBS*.

The farther down the list I read, the more confused I got. Other definitive IBS treatments included (but were certainly not limited to) acupuncture, soluble fiber, herbal remedies, and something called cognitive-behavioral therapy.

I was getting the feeling IBS was a lot like the stock market: nobody had any idea how the thing really worked, but everybody had a theory on how to beat it.

My answer to a better life was somewhere in this list. It had to be. I sized up what I deemed the most promising approaches and bought five books, even laying out the extra cash for next-day delivery.

I vowed to keep trying new approaches until I found the answer. It was simply going to be a process of elimination.

Grounds for Elimination

Dave was trying to put me on the spot, as usual.

"Hey, Timbo, tell these guys those jokes you were telling me the other night."

"No, that's all right," I said.

"Come on," he said. "How does that one go? What has two thumbs, speaks French, and loves blow—"

"That's enough, Dave," I said.

"Let's hear it," Mac said.

I scowled at them and shook my head. "Seriously, not now."

"Wait, Tim doesn't want to tell a joke? Something *must* be wrong," Steve said.

I was in no mood to take center stage, which was too bad because I couldn't have asked for a more captive audience.

They call it a funitel: with seating for twelve and standing room for about twelve more, this enclosed lift whisks skiers and snowboarders to Squaw Valley's best terrain in about ten minutes. From the outside, it looks like somebody took a hundred Super Shuttle vans and fastened them to a continuously moving clothesline hundreds of feet above the ground.

If Dave, Mac, Steve, and I had had the funitel to ourselves, I would have recited every last joke I could remember, if for no other reason than to distract myself for the remainder of what already felt like an interminable ride.

Among those sharing our cramped pod were four teenage snowboard punks listening to their Walkmans at earsplitting volume, a forty-something mom with twin toddler boys clad in protective racing helmets, and a reserved elderly couple.

And, for the first time since we'd started coming to Lake Tahoe three years earlier for our annual guys' weekend, we also had a woman with us.

Erin, a blond, free-spirited girl bursting with energy, was Dave's yoga instructor, interior decorator, and platonic friend. My infatuation with Erin had begun the night before when, seconds after arriving at the cabin, she'd joined us in the hot tub in her bikini. Staying up after everyone else had gone to bed, we'd talked and flirted a little, but that was as far as things had progressed.

My plan was to play it cool for the weekend and ask her out back in San Francisco. In the meantime, I wasn't about to risk blowing my chances with any off-color jokes.

Through the clear Plexiglas, I watched the base lodge and the sprawling parking lot grow smaller and smaller. Two hundred feet above the white, frozen ground, and with another eight minutes left in our ascent, it was a bad time to learn that my latest do-it-yourself project hadn't turned out quite the way I'd hoped.

In one of the IBS books I'd bought, I read about something called visceral hypersensitivity. If I understood the concept correctly, it worked like this: In much the same way that the unstable ground beneath my Marina apartment was overly susceptible to even the earth's most minor tremors, people with IBS have digestive tracts that are noticeably more sensitive to innocuous triggers that most people wouldn't even notice. These triggers can be psychological or physical. Sometimes they can be both.

Several of my self-help books suggested my symptoms would improve if I gave up caffeine. Not only do drinks like coffee irritate the digestive tract, they also throw the central nervous system into hyperdrive, making people overly alert and anxious. I knew all too well that the more anxious I became, the more urgently I had to go—and vice versa. Because caffeine served to turbocharge both ends of the equation, whipping this already vicious circle into a devastating twister, removing it was the key to weakening the storm.

So, without any hesitation, I'd stopped drinking coffee—and soft drinks, too. I'd endured the incessant withdrawal headaches and had struggled through hour after hour of narcoleptic existence. I'd even trained myself to embrace peppermint herbal tea as my new morning beverage of choice.

Over the previous five weeks, I'd attributed my lack of symptoms to my lack of caffeine. Blinded by optimism, I had overlooked some relevant facts. Work had been slow—I hadn't been in a meeting, on a plane, or even stuck in traffic in weeks. My dating life had been just as quiet. So had I been feeling better because I was avoiding caffeine … or had my symptoms disappeared because my life had recently been devoid of the stressful situations that usually triggered my symptoms—like being trapped in this cramped, claustrophobic funitel?

It was now apparent my bowels and nerves didn't need caffeine to stir them into a circular frenzy.

Steve would understand what I was going through, but I couldn't say anything in front of everybody. Neither of us was ready to publicly come out of the water closet.

Instead I looked over at him, using my eyes and my facial muscles to tap out an SOS.

Steve stared back, puzzled by my maniacal facial contortions.

I tried again, widening, narrowing, and then widening my eyeballs. When that didn't work, I cast my eyes downward, toward my stomach this time. He still wasn't picking up on my clues. It was like a bad game of charades.

That was when the loud blast echoed through the funitel. It sounded like an explosion. Even the snowboarders heard it over their music.

"Oh my God, what *was* that?" Erin shouted. I could almost see her heart pounding through her jacket.

All eyes swiveled toward the explosion, which sounded like it had come from a not-too-distant ridge.

I seized the opportunity to kick Steve in the shin and point to my gut.

Now he understood. He turned around to see how much farther we had to go before reaching the top. It wasn't encouraging. Assuming the lift didn't break down, we were looking at another five minutes—an eternity to me. Steve shot me a sympathetic smile and crossed his fingers. I was still freaking out, but knowing I had one person who wouldn't judge me helped lower my anxiety level a notch or two.

Dave explained what was going on: "It's just avalanche blasting. No big deal."

Having feared being thrown out of a Super Shuttle van for fouling the air, I wondered how the strangers in the funitel might react. Surely the snowboarders, who already had chips on their shoulders anyway, possessed enough cumulative muscle to pry the sealed doors open. I glanced out the window. From this height, death was a certainty.

As the seconds crept by, my thoughts turned to my Gore-Tex ski pants. That they were both black and waterproof offered some solace in the event of an accident. Would they be able to keep that kind of odor from breaching the communal air until we reached the summit?

"What do you mean, avalanche blasting?" Erin asked.

Dave loved putting his knowledge of obscure technical matters on display. "After the mountain gets dumped with new snow, like last night, the ski patrol brings out a big artillery gun—an Army 105-millimeter Howitzer, actually—and fires explosive shells at the mountain to start an avalanche."

"Why would they want to start an avalanche on purpose? That sounds dangerous," she said.

"Actually," Dave responded, "it's more dangerous to let the snow build up because it becomes unstable. When it's unstable, you never know when tons of snow might come crashing down the mountain and bury everything in its path. Setting off an intentional avalanche *before* they let skiers onto that part of the mountain actually makes the mountain safer for everyone. Get it?"

As the funitel cleared Squaw's steep granite face, the summit came into view. With relief in sight and no more than a minute and a half away, my sense of urgency eased just enough to give me the confidence that today would not be the day I tested the odor-containing properties of my Gore-Tex pants.

Erin nodded. "Got it."

In one of those "aha" moments, I got it, too.

◆   ◆   ◆

"I'm sorry to have to do this so early, but I've got a lot to do before Monday," she said. "I don't know if I told you, but next week is spring break, and I'm headed off to Belize to go scuba diving."

Her name was Abbey. She taught nursery school over in Marin. We'd met at Cozmo's, a bar up on Chestnut Street, a few weeks after I'd gotten back from skiing in Tahoe.

"Really?" I said. "That sounds so cool. I'd love to do something like that." What I really meant to say was I'd love it if my brain and my digestive tract could get in sync long enough to let me even entertain the idea of taking such an adventurous vacation.

"I'm so excited. It's going to be a blast!" she said. "But enough about me. How's your day going?"

She had no way of knowing that meeting for coffee at Starbucks at eight o'clock on Saturday morning was my idea of the first date from hell. The fact that I was there at all was a testament to the sad state of my dating life.

"So far, so good," I said, yawning and removing sleep from my eyes.

"Well, it looks like somebody's still sleepy. Since I got you out of bed *soooo early*, the first round is on me," Abbey said, her voice heavy with sarcasm. Before I could protest, she had already bounded up to the counter. I stayed behind and held our table.

Unbeknownst to her, I'd been up—intentionally—since the uncivilized hour of 5:45 for the sole purpose of preparing for our eight o'clock date. That's when I'd thrown on my jeans, sweater, and baseball hat and had driven up to the Coffee Roastery on Chestnut Street.

After the funitel ride in Tahoe, I had begun to look at coffee in a whole new light. The way I saw it, each morning my colon contained the equivalent of at least three feet, maybe four, of freshly fallen snow. Though the plan initially seemed counterintuitive, wouldn't it make sense to begin each day by taking aim at this unstable mass with my own Howitzer shell—a piping-hot cup of coffee? Even if this personal avalanche blasting couldn't shake loose every last piece of threatening loose matter, surely it would cause most of my bulk to fall safely out of harm's way.

"I'll have a double espresso and …" Abbey's raspy voice carried across the room, even cutting through the high-pitched squeals of the cappuccino machine. She was no mousey nursery-school teacher. She turned and shouted, "Tim, how about you? Do you want a double espresso?"

"No, thanks … I'll have … um …"

As with fire, harsh penalties await those who don't respect coffee's raw, unforgiving power. Thanks to my predawn drive to the Coffee Roastery, my avalanche blasting was already done for the day. I'd made my slopes as safe as they were going to be. Nothing good could come from further blasting.

"Regular coffee?" she shouted again. "Cappuccino?"

Once the avalanche blasting was done for the day, you had to put the Howitzer away.

"No, I think I'll have …"

Whatever you do, do not *touch the Howitzer.*

"Don't even tell me you're a latte guy," she yelled.

Does she have to shout this out for public consumption? I could swear her voice was getting louder and more disapproving each time she interrupted me. Now people were staring. The barista behind the counter, the customers in line, and even the tourists sitting at the next table seemed to be waiting for my reply. Would I admit, they must have wondered, to being a latte guy?

"Come on, are you joking?" I said. "No way."

She looked relieved.

"How about some herbal tea?" I asked. "Do they have peppermint?"

Abbey walked over with our drinks, handing me my caffeine-free peppermint tea.

"Wow, this is a first," she said. "I've never met a guy who drinks herbal tea before. Don't you like coffee?"

Was it my imagination or was this nursery-school teacher calling my masculinity into question based on my beverage choice? What was the big deal about herbal tea?

"No, I do," I said. "A lot, actually."

But, I wondered, what if I didn't? Where was it written you were not a real man if you didn't drink coffee? And if she felt this way about coffee, how would she react if I told her almost every decision I made revolved around being near a bathroom?

"Uh-huh. Sure," she said. I could tell she didn't believe me.

"Really, I already had two cups earlier this morning. One more might put me over the edge. I'm being serious."

I found myself on the receiving end of a look that Abbey no doubt reserved for five-year-olds who told tall tales. "If you say so," she said.

Abbey's attitude was getting under my skin. We were only ten minutes into our first date, and from where I sat, things weren't going so well. In a last-ditch effort to shift gears and get onto a new topic, I asked her to tell me about her job.

She talked about the joys of teaching nursery school and how her students just lit up whenever she read Dr. Seuss.

"*Green Eggs and Ham* is their favorite," she said.

As I pretended to listen, I silently set about explaining my relationship with coffee in terms Abbey might understand.

I'll always drink it in the morning, before six or eight
But never, never will I drink coffee on a date.

I'll always drink some at home, and maybe on a train
But never, never will I drink coffee on a plane.

Because the huge brown stain would look tacky
Never, never will I drink coffee while wearing khaki.

Because my bowel control can be fleeting
I refuse to sip coffee during a meeting.

I have no problem with apple pie à la mode
But I won't dare drink coffee if I'm far from a commode.

Bumper-to-bumper traffic makes my stomach hyper
But add a few sips of coffee, and I'm gonna need a diaper.

In no uncertain terms, let me give you the scoop
I only drink coffee if I know there's a place where I can poop.

After a half hour, we parted ways with a handshake. Abbey flew off to Belize to add more adventure to her life, while I stayed put and redoubled my efforts to reduce the adventure in mine.

◆   ◆   ◆

Paul walked right past my desk and headed toward the door.

I had to shout. "What? You're not even going to ask me?"

My new boss spun around in slow motion, bewildered. "You're kidding, right?"

"No, I'm not," I said.

He looked as if he wanted to strangle me. Instead he couldn't help but laugh at the obvious absurdity of the situation.

"You swear you're not messing with me?" Paul asked. "You *really* want to go?"

"I do, I swear."

"Well, then, by all means. I'd be honored by your presence," he said, shaking his head in confusion. I'd been working at LPM for two months. Every day Paul had asked me to join him on his midmorning coffee jaunt. Every day I had said no. Until today.

Outside our office on the ninth floor, we waited. It was an old building with five old elevators that kept us waiting, no matter what time of day.

"So, I'm curious. Why today?" Paul asked.

"I don't know why," I said. "I just felt like taking a break and getting some fresh air, I guess."

Really, it was just plain stupid to pass up opportunities to bond with my boss. As usual, the elevator stopped on all but one floor during what felt like a three-minute ride to the lobby.

Paul was a workaholic, but not by choice. Forty years old with a stay-at-home wife, two young kids, and an overpriced waterfront home in chichi Tiburon, he'd become a slave to making enough money to continue living the upmarket lifestyle he had doggedly created for himself.

Once outside we walked to the corner of Montgomery and Pine, where we missed our turn in the crosswalk by two seconds. Next to the elevator ride that lowered me from the safety of the ninth floor men's room down to the hostile, foreign land below, I always hated waiting at the crosswalks the most.

I knew it took a full two minutes for the traffic lights to cycle through their preprogrammed sequence. For 120 anxious seconds, I was vulnerable, a fact that made every trip to get lunch, get my haircut, or go to the dentist all the more terrifying. Unlike most Californians, I rarely passed up an opportunity to jaywalk. Unfortunately this was a busy intersection.

The Financial District didn't have any gas stations to pop into, only tall buildings, most of whose lobbies offered no place for weary pedestrians to relieve themselves. The Hotel Mandarin, two blocks away, was an exception.

As was my habit, I continued to count the seconds down—silently, of course. *Sixty-two, sixty-one, sixty ... OK, halfway. Almost there.*

As the steady stream of cars, trucks, and buses barreled down Montgomery Street, continuing to impede our swift crossing, Paul said, "So how's your presentation coming along? I noticed that you've been spending a lot of time working on it."

Forty-nine, forty-eight, forty-seven ... Would it be quicker to take the elevator back up to the ninth floor, or hustle over to the Mandarin? I mean, if I had to—which I don't. Not yet. But what if I did have to, in an emergency? Forty, thirty-nine, thirty-eight ...

"The presentation's coming along pretty well, thanks. I think I'm finally getting comfortable with it. Obviously, I'll have a better answer for you after next week."

Thirty-one, thirty, twenty-nine ... You got it. Nothing to worry about. You're in the homestretch. Twenty-four, twenty-three, twenty-two ...

"Oh, that's right. Your first big trip without the training wheels," Paul said, referring to the fact that until then, I'd been joining Paul on his sales calls so I could learn the ropes. "Where are you off to?"

Five, four, three ...

"Iowa," I said.

We walked into the Bank of America building's concourse and got in line at Starbucks.

After visualizing the journey to Iowa that awaited me, I said, "I hope this lead turns out to be worth the trip."

"Hey," Paul said, "you never know until you get there."

If getting on a plane gave Paul even the most remote chance to close a deal and earn a commission check, he was all over it. Even if it was a long shot, Paul never hesitated to jump on a 5:00 AM flight to the middle of nowhere to "run out the ground ball," as he liked to say. I'm sure that was what he expected from me when he hired me.

"And remember," Paul added, "my W-2 is tied to your W-2." He was fond of reminding me in a lighthearted tone that since he was my manager, the more I made, the more he made. And conversely, the less I made, the less he made. He was kind of kidding … but not really.

We took a seat on a nearby bench, sipped our coffee, and continued chatting.

Despite the fact that the concourse had no public restrooms—not even at Starbucks—I wasn't preoccupied with sprinting over to the Hotel Mandarin, calculating how long it would take to navigate my way back across Montgomery Street, or predicting the improbable odds of a speedy elevator ride back up to the ninth floor. For once I enjoyed a rare luxury: listening without distraction. It was an incredible glimpse into a state of mind I assumed most everybody in the world took for granted.

The source of my calmness—a plastic card that had arrived in the mail a day earlier—sat in my front left pocket, tucked securely into the sterling-silver billfold that Cynthia had given to me for Christmas.

In a timely promotional offer, the Bay Club, the gym I belonged to but rarely used, had recently invited me to upgrade to an executive membership that would give me access to their other location in the city. Even though I could barely justify the cost of *one* gym, I jumped at their invitation to pay an extra $45 each month to join a second one. The location was too convenient to pass up.

Twenty yards from Starbucks and the bench where Paul and I sipped our coffee, just on the other side of the smoked-glass doors that coldly proclaimed "Bay Club—Members Only," was a wide array of state-of-the-art fitness machines that I would never use … and more important, a men's locker room with four toilets I couldn't live without.

In this inhospitable land without toilets, I now had the shelter of an embassy.

On one level, it was a form of salvation, but on another level, I felt like a coward. Rather than facing down my fears, had I simply opted to take the easy way out by buying a crutch? Even though I had no idea how to counter my fears, would giving in to them only reinforce them?

These were questions I would have plenty of time to ponder while calmly waiting in line for my grande drip coffee at Starbucks ... or while flying to Iowa, where there were no Bay Clubs.

Bulking Up

"You know her?"

"Yeah, her name's Wendy," Elise said. "I've met her of a bunch of times. Sweet girl."

To gain insight into the female psyche, something I tried to do pretty much all the time, I relied on a three-prong strategy: watch *Sex and the City* each week (even the reruns were instructive), read at least two issues of *Cosmopolitan* per year, and consult my trusted personal dating advisor—Elise.

As longtime friends and co-workers back at Robertson Stephens, Elise and I had racked up hundreds of hours attempting to demystify the baffling behavior of our respective genders to one another. Most of the time, we talked strategy. "How long should I wait to call her?" Or, "It's been four days … why hasn't he called me back?"

Now Elise and I had been reunited at LPM. Paul had let us arrange our desks directly opposite one another, and each day we would sit down and face each other in the same way as two people sitting across from one another at a picnic table. In fact, there was no shortage of slow periods—sometimes days in a row—when our Siamese desks became exactly that—a picnic table.

Over long breakfasts and even longer lunches eaten at our desks (leaving for lunch hour implied a substandard work ethic), we would discuss such topics as my never-ending dating dramas, her addiction to ridiculously expensive brands like Prada and Gucci, and our frustration over the likelihood that no matter how successful we became, we would never be able to afford to buy homes in San Francisco.

"Is she … you know …"

"Yes, Tim, she's very pretty. And smart, too. She's a lawyer."

Allison, a former co-worker, had left me a voice mail saying she wanted to set me up with her sister, Wendy, who had recently broken up with her boyfriend.

"Do you think I'm her type?" I asked Elise.

"I'm not sure. She's really cool, but she's a little bit of a tomboy. I kind of picture her with a man's man."

"So, what do you think?" I asked. "I'm a man's man, right?"

When Paul walked by, our spoken conversation shifted to e-mail. Elise hit the keyboard without missing a beat.

I clicked on my inbox. Elise's answer: "Mmm … I think so. More or less."

What is she talking about? I tapped out an angry reply: *"Huh?"*

Elise's expression turned pensive as she crafted her response. I hit Refresh five times before her reply popped up on my screen.

"Don't take this the wrong way. The triathlon stuff is very manly. But the fact that you used to shave your legs and don't follow professional sports is a little suspect. Also, it wouldn't kill you to hit the weight room. You could use a little more bulk."

There was that word again: *bulk.* This was the second time in twenty-four hours someone had advised me to bulk up.

When I called Allison back later that day, I had a whole slew of questions. For starters, what part of town did Wendy live in? Was she really as much of a tomboy as Elise thought she was?

Allison sounded perplexed with my line of questioning. "Well, she just bought a house over in the Haight, but the street she lives on is pretty safe. And yes, she's really into sports, especially baseball. She even has season tickets for the Oakland A's. What guy wouldn't love that?"

Trying to ascertain what kind of guys Wendy typically dated, I inquired as tactfully as I could about her most recent boyfriend. "It's not that I'm insecure. I just want to make sure we're compatible. You understand."

"He's in the navy," Allison said without elaboration.

"Oh, really? Does he wear one of those little sailor suits?"

"God, no," she said. "He's a pilot … flies F-14s."

Yikes! Wendy's last boyfriend defended his country by flying supersonic combat jets off of aircraft carriers. Now her sister was trying to fix her up with a guy who would have to muster up all his courage just to drive to the other side of San Francisco to pick her up for a date.

"Well, that's a relief," I said. "For a second, I thought I might be following in the footsteps of some kind of total stud."

"Oh, give me a break," Allison said. "My sister likes confident, take-charge guys. You have nothing to worry about. Just be yourself. Oh, and call her soon. She's waiting."

◆   ◆   ◆

It had been an exhilarating day, and I just couldn't keep it to myself. Driving back from my meeting in Berkeley, I picked up my cell phone and called my boss.

"Hello, you've reached the voice mail for Paul …"

Damn.

"Hey, Paul, I'm just calling to let you know my meetings went really well today. All my practice is paying off. I nailed the presentation. I'll see you in the office tomorrow."

Now I felt as if I had redeemed myself, at least partially. At any rate, this was a nice recovery from Iowa, where a sudden onset of rectal urgency had led me to cancel one of my two meetings at the last minute. I'd told Paul it had been the prospect who'd canceled the meeting, not me.

"Hey, that kind of thing happens from time to time. Some people are just inconsiderate," he'd told me. "Don't let it frustrate you too much."

His pep talk had made me feel like even more of a weasel.

But today I hadn't had to cancel anything. Feeling proud of having put in a hard, honest day's work, I headed back home. Anticipating that Wendy would agree to at least one date, I had decided bulking up would be a good idea after all. I would start immediately.

I had no intention of going to either of my gyms, no plan to pump iron, and no desire to increase the size of my physical frame. No, my regimen would be as effortless as opening the economy-sized cylinder of Metamucil I'd just bought in Berkeley, stirring a few tablespoons into a tall glass of water, and doing some good, old-fashioned six-ounce curls.

On the surface, treating my overproductive digestive tract with a known laxative sounded about as smart as using Drano to fix a leaking pipe. But my IBS books insisted fiber's bulking properties made it an ideal tool for treating constipation *and* diarrhea.

At around four o'clock, I breezed through the toll plaza and accelerated onto the upper deck of the Bay Bridge. Hurtling unimpeded toward San Francisco along the bridge's five-mile span, I thanked my lucky stars that for the second time today, I was traveling in the opposite direction of the commuting masses.

I was still trying to figure out how fiber would benefit my overproductive bowels when I realized the answer was right in front of me. As best I could tell, my digestive tract resembled the Bay Bridge's endless stream of random cars and trucks racing willy-nilly toward San Francisco. Fiber would make it operate more like the BART train, which gathered up all the stray commuters and transported them safely to the station on a predictable, published schedule.

Still buzzing with confidence from my meetings, I decided it was the perfect time to call Wendy. I didn't feel the least bit nervous as I dialed her number. *So what if she dated a fighter pilot? I'm a goddamned investment salesman with a great job, a brand-new Audi, and a sweet apartment!* No small talk, I decided. No beating around the bush. When she answered, I would jump right in and take charge.

She picked up on the second ring, her high-pitched, feminine voice inviting yet professional. "Hello, this is Wendy."

"Hi, Wendy. It's Tim Phelan." Brief. Firm. Masculine.

"Hi, Tim. My sister said you'd be calling."

"So, what do you say we get together? Are you free next Friday night?"

"As a matter of fact, I am."

"Great. I'll make a reservation."

"Hey, if you're up for it, I've been dying to try this new restaurant. I can't remember the name of it, but it's over in the East Bay ... in Berkeley, I think. Oh, what's it called? Give me a second, I'll think of it ..."

Still speeding toward San Francisco on the Bay Bridge's upper deck, I was all too aware of the hell that was playing out on the bridge's lower deck, the one that led commuters away from the city and back to their homes in the East Bay each evening. It was jam-packed with vehicles traveling slower than most people walked.

On a good day, the bumper-to-bumper traffic below showed no signs of easing until eight or nine o'clock at night. But, of course, throw one stalled car or a jumper threatening suicide into the mix (both occurred with alarming frequency), and all bets were off. I knew people who had been stuck on this bridge for five or six hours at a time.

It didn't matter what the name of that restaurant was because there was no way in hell I was going to subject myself to crossing that bridge with the rest of the world during primetime. Not next Friday night, or the Friday night after that, either.

"Actually, I already had a place in mind," I said. *That's it. Be a leader. Take charge.* "It's near my apartment in the Marina. Café Marimba."

"I heard that's supposed to be really good," Wendy said. "I've never been there."

"Me neither," I claimed. "It'll be fun to check it out."

"Tell you what," Wendy said, "since I live on the other side of town, I think it makes sense if I drive over and meet you there. I mean, if that's OK with you."

She wasn't even going to make me pick her up? What had I possibly done to deserve *this* kind of luck? I liked her already.

"I suppose I can live with that," I said. "But you have to promise not to give me a hard time for shirking my responsibilities as a gentleman."

"Provided you promise to behave like a perfect gentleman for the rest of the night, then you've got a deal," she said, speaking like a true attorney.

"I can't guarantee anything, but I promise to try."

"Fair enough," she said.

I knew I couldn't avoid driving to Wendy's house, or the East Bay, forever. Like Cynthia, Wendy was bound to have her breaking point. I looked over at the tube of Metamucil riding shotgun in my passenger seat. I didn't want to get my hopes too high, but if adding bulk could give me the kind of regularity I'd been led to believe it could, then maybe I would actually be able to drive across this bridge, just like the brave commuters on the lower deck ... just like a normal human being.

◆   ◆   ◆

Thanks to two pitchers of margaritas, the restaurant's dual restrooms, and the close proximity to my apartment, my first date with Wendy had been a big success.

Yes, Wendy was obsessed with professional baseball, and yes, she was a hard-charging prosecutor, but she was also a sweet, genuine person. She'd never once missed an opportunity to pass along a heartfelt "please" or "thank you" to the restaurant's staff. Even the busboy had received a beaming smile and a friendly "*gracias.*" *This has promise*, I thought.

Two weeks later, I drove up to Tahoe to meet Wendy at her sister's ski cabin.

The first morning when I walked into the bathroom, Wendy was there, brushing her teeth.

"Oh, sorry, I didn't know you were in here."

"Do you need to use the bathroom?" she asked.

"Um, I do. But I can wait."

"Go ahead. I don't mind," Wendy said.

I didn't want to rush her—it looked like she was close to finishing anyway. I leaned against the wall and waited. She looked at me, confused as to why I wasn't going about my business. Now *I* was confused.

"Uhhh, yeah … well … the thing is … what I need to do is *not* … you know …" —I pointed my index fingers clumsily toward my fly—"*pee*."

She didn't even blink. "Yeah, I get it. So what? My old boyfriend and I used to sit on the toilet in front of each other all the time. Seriously, it's no big deal."

Uh-huh. Right.

"Really?" I asked.

She nodded. "Really."

I waited for her to burst out laughing and shout, "Just kidding!" I was thrilled she didn't have any hang-ups about bodily functions, but I still wasn't ready for things to move this quickly. I never would have dreamed of doing this in front of Cynthia. And Wendy and I hadn't even been on six dates.

"I … I … uuhh … no … can't … sorry," I stammered. "I mean I'm just … not exactly … comf … comfort … comfortable … doing … uh, well … *that* … in front of you. Sorry."

"Tim, listen," she said. "I don't want to make you feel uncomfortable. If you want to use the bathroom in private, go right ahead. All I'm saying is I'm not squeamish about that stuff." Then she smiled, kissed me on my lips, and turned to walk out of the bathroom.

"Thank you," I said.

Then I locked the door.

I must have been on the toilet for twenty minutes, but I couldn't help it. I'd been using the Metamucil for three weeks. Religiously. Every day. And so far, it hadn't done the trick. For starters, I had *lots* of gas—a situation the high altitude only aggravated. Worse, the Metamucil was acting more like fertilizer, sending me to the bathroom more often than ever. Thinking maybe it would just take more time, I stuck with it.

That afternoon, when Wendy was taking a nap and Allison and her husband were at the supermarket, I slipped into the empty kitchen. After filling a tumbler with cold water, I began to extract the fiber from the massive plastic container, which towered over the Formica counter as inconspicuously as the Empire State Building over Manhattan.

Fiber, I'd learned, was all about precision. Too much or too little could have disastrous consequences. So I examined each spoonful closely to make sure it was the same size as the last. The first scoop was perfect; I dumped it into the waiting tumbler. Removing the second load from the container, I raised the spoon up to my eyes to get a closer look. I was so focused on the exact height of the orange fiber crystals in the spoon that I didn't immediately see I was no longer alone.

Standing directly in front of me, no more than three feet away, was Wendy. Busted. She'd been watching for at least a minute.

First the twenty-minute toilet session. Now this midafternoon fiber cocktail. She didn't have to be a lawyer to see something unusual was afoot.

"What are you doing?" she asked.

All of a sudden, for no good reason, I felt as if I were being cross-examined on the witness stand. *Do you swear to tell the truth, the whole truth, and nothing but the truth, so help you God?*

"I've been having some digestive troubles recently," I said, "and I read this is supposed to help."

But that was *all* I told her. I saw no need to mention the restrictive anxieties or the immobilizing phobias that stemmed from my digestive troubles … no need to raise a red flag and scare anybody by throwing the phrase *irritable bowel* around the cabin.

On our last day at Tahoe, my honesty was tested yet again, along with my courage. We met up with a bunch of Wendy's friends for a day of skiing at North Star. Seeing the only way to get to the top of the mountain was by riding in an enclosed gondola half the size of the dreaded funitel over at Squaw Valley, I told Wendy everyone should go ahead without me.

"Is this about your stomach problems?" she asked.

"Well, my stomach still isn't feeling that great," I said. "But it has more to do with being claustrophobic. I don't like small spaces."

I didn't mind if Wendy thought I was claustrophobic—lots of people were. And I didn't mind if she thought I had digestive troubles—again, lots of people did. I just didn't feel comfortable admitting the two were linked.

"You're claustrophobic?" she asked. "Honestly?"

"I'm afraid so," I said.

Taking the news in stride, Wendy said, "I can always see my friends another time. The only thing that would upset me was if I didn't get to spend the day with you."

Did she really feel this way? Maybe not, but I chose to believe her, essentially giving myself a permission slip to continue to put my fears in front of her desires. She'd understand, right?

Yes, of course she would.

◆　　◆　　◆

"I still have time to go to the men's room, don't I?"

Wendy looked at her watch and then up at me. "How badly do you have to go?"

I mulled over how to best phrase my answer. "Let's put it this way. There's no way I'll be able to wait until the intermission."

For Valentine's Day, Wendy had surprised me with two tickets for *Defending the Caveman*, a comical one-man show about the differences between men and women.

She flipped through the playbill. "Actually, then you better go now," she said. "This show doesn't have an intermission."

I couldn't believe what I'd just heard. "You've *got* to be kidding me. What kind of show doesn't have an intermission? The damn thing is close to two hours long, and there's no frigging break? What the hell do they expect people to ..."

Even before this outburst, Wendy must have started to wonder about me. When she had first phoned to tell me about the tickets, my reaction should have been to say something along the lines of, "That's so thoughtful. Thank you. What a fun way to spend Valentine's Day."

Instead I'd hit her with the usual rapid-fire interrogation. *Where is the theater? What time is the show? Where are our seats? How close to the stage are they? Will we be sitting on an aisle? Are you sure our seats aren't in the middle of a row? Are you positive?*

"Sssshhh!" Wendy said with her finger to her mouth, looking around the theater. "Could you please lower your voice?"

"I'm sorry. You're right," I whispered. "I just know I won't be able to hold it in for two hours."

She looked at me like I was insane. "Who said you have to?"

"What do you mean? You can't leave your seat during the performance. It's against the rules."

Now she was trying not to laugh. "Against the rules? You obviously haven't spent much time at the theater. Trust me: people get up and leave their seats all the time. It's perfectly fine."

In the interest of time, I chose not to argue. "You know more about this than I do, but I'm still going to make a quick trip."

God, I wanted to believe her, but I couldn't bring myself to trust her on this one. A recent trip with my mom to the symphony had taught me otherwise. It was bad enough the audience had been reminded to refrain from talking and moving, but I'd been blown away at the sight of ushers marching down the aisles passing out cough drops. *They don't even want you to cough?* Clearly the symphony was no place for a guy like me.

I walked back from the men's room and took my seat. The lights went down. The curtain came up. Then, right before my very eyes, there he was: the caveman.

Right away I could tell he was the epitome of a man's man. An ordinary-looking guy in his late thirties or early forties, he was dressed in jeans, sneakers, and an untucked T-shirt. He sported a modest beer gut and carried a spear.

His opening lines were so hysterical that for a few wonderful minutes, I forgot all about how my bulking-up regimen hadn't yet cured me.

It wasn't long before the distraction wore off, and I scanned the theater. I glanced over toward the center rows and then behind me, looking back at the people seated between me and the lobby.

So far nobody had gotten up. I looked around again, this time up to the balcony. I saw nothing, not even an usher escorting late arrivals to their seats. Had Wendy intentionally given me a bum steer so I wouldn't stress out over not having an intermission?

The show had only been going on for about five or six minutes. For the next fifteen, I alternated between howling at the caveman and monitoring the movement—or lack thereof—of the audience. I couldn't relax until I knew it was acceptable for me to walk away if I needed to.

Looking back at the stage, I began to identify even more with the caveman. We had a lot in common, it seemed. He didn't seem like he would associate with the snooty symphony types. He was unpolished and politically incorrect—the kind of guy who would understand that another guy might have to get up to use the toilet.

But if the caveman was my kind of guy, I still considered the rest of the audience suspect.

It wasn't until forty agonizing minutes into the performance that a middle-aged man smack dab in the middle seat of the center row stood up and made twelve or thirteen people to his left retract their knees so he could pass by. Seconds after that brave pioneer made his move, others followed—quickly, and from all directions. I guess nobody else had wanted to be the first, either.

As I stood up and followed suit, I thought that in many ways, it was too bad *I* hadn't been born in the Stone Age, when people lived without the pressure and peering eyes of a well-behaved, judgmental society. Back then there were no elite arbiters of decorum and manners. There was no symphony. No opera. Nobody passed out cough drops. There weren't even any toilets. Cavemen relieved themselves whenever and wherever they damn well felt like it. Period. *You don't like it? Too bad! I'm a caveman, damn it!*

The show, while entertaining, was also painful because it forced me to take an uncomfortable look in the mirror. Onstage was the guy I wanted to be. Underneath my uncontrollable laughter, I was reminded of how far away I actually was.

◆　　◆　　◆

"Do you want to go to the A's game with me tomorrow night?" Wendy asked.

The usual interrogation revealed the Oakland A's were going to play the Baltimore Orioles the following night. The game would start at 7:00 PM, which meant we should plan on leaving by five thirty.

"Are we going to drive?" I asked this as if her answer would help me decide. Whatever our mode of transportation, we still had to cross the bay to get to Oakland. The BART train would take about thirty minutes, but without bathrooms in the trains, that wasn't going to happen. The only other option was the Bay Bridge, which we'd be hitting head-on at the peak of rush hour.

I took Wendy at her word that she didn't have an issue with me going to the bathroom in front of her. As unfathomable as it was to me, she really did seem to mean it. But I was quite certain she was speaking about using an actual toilet—the porcelain kind. While she hadn't come right out and said it, I was pretty sure she would not have been as cool when it came to watching me eliminate my solid waste in the passenger seat of her BMW.

I'd be forced to get out of the car and hang my bare ass hundreds of feet above the water below. Somebody would probably call 911 to report me to the authorities as a jumper. They'd try to talk me down, but by that point, I'd probably consider jumping.

"No, thanks, I'd rather not go," I said. "It's too short of notice, and besides, I'm not much of a baseball fan. It wouldn't be fun for me. You understand, don't you?"

She didn't. What she heard was that I was only willing to participate in activities if they directly interested *me*. Where was my willingness to participate in activities that didn't appeal to me but would make *her* happy? Why couldn't I sacrifice a couple of hours for one night to make my girlfriend happy?

When I declined to explain the real reason, I knew I was pushing my luck. I just didn't know how close I was to reaching her breaking point. It didn't take long after that—only about two weeks—for Wendy to decide our relationship wasn't meeting her needs. "Compatibility issues," she said.

After Wendy broke up with me, I decided it was time to part ways with my Metamucil. It seemed we weren't right for each other, either. My confidence was once again in tatters, and once again I had a lot of free time on my hands. So I decided to head to the gym, where I could bulk up like a real man.

The Human Water Balloon

It was two thirty in the afternoon. If we didn't find something else to talk about, we would have no choice. We would have to go back to work. There was a moment of silence. We looked at each other, knowing what was at stake. One of us needed to come up with a worthy subject.

Elise made the first move. I suppose it was just a matter of time. In seven years, we had exhausted every other conceivable topic. She went right for the elephant in the living room.

"OK, so what's the deal with you and the bathroom?"

Hardball.

"Excuse me?" I asked. I tried to play dumb, but she was way too sharp. Exactly what did she know? Confirming her suspicions was one thing. Freely spilling my guts was something else.

"Well, for starters, I've noticed you make frequent trips down the hall to the men's room … all day long. I've also noticed there's a pattern to your trips … before conference calls, before team meetings, before going out to get lunch, and *always* a few times after your morning Starbucks run."

I was stunned. She was on to me—and probably had been for years. I thought I had kept my little condition secret. I was wrong. Looking Elise in the eye, I opened my mouth … and just froze.

When Elise wanted an answer, she got an answer. "Well, jerky? I asked you a question. What's the deal?"

I proceeded to spend the next ten minutes explaining how my bowels had a long history of rebelling against me at the most inconvenient times. I told her about how they had a mind of their own and could sense when I wasn't near a toilet, picking that precise moment to stage their violent protests. I tried to explain how this unpredictability led to me living in a near-constant state of hypervigilance, and how that anxiety, as best as I could tell, triggered the urgent onset of my symptoms.

She sat on her side of our picnic table and listened. When I had finished my explanation, she smiled, nodded, and said, "Do you know what you need?"

"Potty training?" I whispered, looking around to make sure nobody was tuned in.

"A colonic," she said, just loudly enough to call attention to our discussion.

My only knowledge of colonics came from the movies. In *L.A. Story*, Sarah Jessica Parker's character scheduled one for her date, played by Steve Martin. All I gathered from the context of the scene was that a colonic involved pumping large amounts of fluid into your ass—ostensibly for your health. I remembered wincing in sympathy as Steve Martin emerged from the session and limped down the stairs in obvious discomfort.

"Huh?" I asked.

"No, I'm being serious. I'll bet you probably have some type of bacteria in your intestines or in your colon that's causing your bowel issues. A colonic is designed to go in and clean your pipes out … completely." She wasn't laughing.

"It's sort of like the Roto-Rooter treatment for your digestive system," she added with a smile. "It's safe and healthy. Lots of people use them to cleanse their bodies of toxins. It'll make you feel like a new person."

I asked, "How do you know so much about this, anyway?"

She turned away and began to type on her keyboard. *She's blowing me off, isn't she?* I repeated my question. Again she offered no response, continuing to type away. *Great, I tell her my secret, and she gives me nothing in return. That's the last time I share something personal with her.*

Two seconds later, an e-mail popped onto my screen. It was from Elise. It was a link to the Web site of a company called Inner-Gize. Elise leaned across the desk and whispered, "Tell 'em I sent you."

❖   ❖   ❖

Inner-Gize had an opening the following afternoon. This was great because I wouldn't have time to worry about it or chicken out. Unfortunately I'd scheduled a date for that evening.

What kind of physical condition would I be in after my Roto-Rooter appointment? I remembered my enema disaster in the Super Shuttle years earlier. Those aftershocks had continued for hours—and that was just an enema. A colonic would be like a supersized, industrial-strength enema. It might be days before I could safely venture outside my apartment.

At a recent dinner party, I'd unexpectedly bumped into Erin, Dave's friend whom I'd met in Tahoe. Like me, she was currently single. Would she remember the chemistry we both felt that night when I stayed up and watched TV with her? Was it too late to rekindle it? It was worth a shot, I'd decided.

I'd been looking forward to taking her out all week, and I didn't want to postpone our first official date. I also didn't want to run the risk of having any unanticipated physical side effects from the colonic mess up our evening.

TMI stands for "too much information." In the dating world, providing your date with TMI too soon could be grounds for immediate dismissal. Would discussing the fact that I believed I suffered from irritable bowel syndrome qualify as TMI? Absolutely.

Would telling Erin before our first date that I was voluntarily going to undergo a hydrocolonic therapy session count as TMI? Well, if we were in Southern California, probably not. In San Francisco, it was a toss-up. It wasn't worth the risk. My challenge was going to be to postpone the date without being too specific about why. I picked up the phone.

"Hey, Tim. What's up?"

"Not much. Listen, I was calling to talk to you about tomorrow night."

"Oh, I haven't forgotten," she said. "What do you have in mind? Sushi? How about Thai food?"

"Well, actually ..." I paused. "I've got a little bit of a problem with tomorrow night. I hate to say it, but I think we might have to reschedule for next week."

"Are you kidding me? Why? Do you have to work?" She wasn't happy about this change of plans.

"No, it's not work. It's ... well, kind of a medical thing," I said, trying to sound as vague and nonspecific as possible. "I'm not sick. I just have to go in for a little procedure tomorrow afternoon, and I'm not really sure how I'm going to feel afterward. I might be fine, but I don't know for sure, and I don't want to ruin our date. Does that make sense?"

I thought I had given out the optimal amount of information—not TMI and not TLI (too little information).

"Exactly what kind of procedure are you going in for?" She wasn't about to let me off the hook without a thorough explanation.

This wasn't going so well. I had painted myself into a corner. *Should I lie? Should I throw her a few additional morsels of information, hoping that she'll be satisfied?* I panicked.

Part of me wanted to tell her everything. I was tired of keeping my condition a secret from people, especially the women I wanted to date. Living a lie was hard work. Why couldn't we live in a world where discussing bodily functions didn't carry such a stigma?

As I continued my descent down this slippery slope, I contemplated the consequences of revealing the details of the colonic and my bowel dysfunction to Erin at such an early stage.

Still painfully aware that not coming clean had cost me my relationship with Wendy, I considered what might happen if I wasn't forthcoming with Erin. I certainly didn't want to make *that* mistake again. Elise had been totally cool about it; maybe Erin would be, too.

After all, when I met her in Tahoe, it was obvious she had a great sense of humor and was not easily offended. If she could endure a weekend as the only woman in a ski house full of belching, farting, and obscenity-spewing men, she might just be cool enough to take news like this in stride. As if walking over thin ice, I proceeded with caution, one small step at a time.

"What kind of procedure? Well, it's a little awkward to talk about. It's kind of embarrassing," I blurted out, continuing to give her more rope to hang me with.

"Listen, my dad's a doctor, and I'm used to hearing about this kind of stuff," Erin said. "Whatever it is, it's no big deal to me, OK? Is it sexual? It's an STD, isn't it? You have herpes, don't you? No, wait, is it plastic surgery? Are you having excessive back hair removed?"

Compared to what Erin's imagination was coming up with, a colonic didn't seem so terrible. It was time to come clean and take my chances. I told her I had a history of chronic digestive issues and that out of desperation, I was exploring alternative treatments—thus the colonic. Her reaction surprised me.

"So you're getting a colonic. Why does that embarrass you? Who gives a shit?" she said, then laughed at her own joke.

We both started to laugh. This woman was pretty cool. I liked her sense of humor, but I couldn't let her show me up.

"Hey, shit happens, right?" I said. More laughter.

"Yeah, but the shit better not hit the fan," she said.

"Well, I'd offer to take you out tomorrow, but it would probably just be the same shit, different day," I shot back.

"Fuck that shit!" was Erin's best response.

We were both giggling like second graders using profanity for the first time. After the laughter subsided, I felt much more comfortable with the thought of going out with Erin under less-than-ideal conditions. If I did have a close call or an accident, I imagined we would end up just laughing it off … after cleaning up, of course.

"Erin, you know what? Why don't we just go ahead and see each other tomorrow night? If you're cool with it, then I'm cool with it. My only request is that we stay in the neighborhood, just in case some shit goes down," I said. "That way, I won't be …"

"Shit out of luck? Up Shit Creek?" she said. We had finally exhausted the depths of our fecal idioms.

"Great. I'll pick you up at seven," I said. "What's your apartment number?"

Apparently she wasn't quite done yet.

"Number *two!*" she howled.

As I hung up the phone, she was still laughing.

◆   ◆   ◆

I was nervous, hopeful, and desperate. I got off the elevator five minutes early at 3:55 and found the Inner-Gize suite. The sign on the door said: "Session in progress. Please do not disturb."

So I did what I always do when I had five minutes to kill before an appointment. Out of habit, I searched for the men's room. Why did I feel the need to empty my bowels just moments before I was going to pay good money to have somebody do it for me? I didn't know. But I had always tidied up my apartment *before* the maid showed up. Go figure.

At first glance, the reception room looked more like a psychedelic opium den. It had a New Age look and feel, but delivered with New Economy efficiency. I heard soothing chanting music—from the digital CD sound system with five-disc carousel in Dolby surround sound. I saw several miniature Buddha statues—standing right next to a twenty-one-inch Sony flat-screen color monitor. I noticed little packets of natural herbs spread out in display in front of the receptionist's desk—presumably for sale because they were located right next to the Visa/MasterCard electronic swipe terminal.

I'd grown up in the suburbs. I shopped at Brooks Brothers. This was definitely not my scene.

"Hi, you must be Tim," the woman behind the desk said. "This is your first visit, right?" She handed me a clipboard and a pen. "This is our legal disclosure that we have all of our patients read and sign, OK?"

OK.

As I read, I saw something I didn't understand. I reread the paragraph. Twice. "Certified Hydrocolonic Technician (CHT)" referred to the qualifications of the person who would be performing this highly invasive procedure, and it was a term I was unfamiliar with. Sorry, but I needed some clarification on this one.

"Excuse me, but I'm a little confused," I said. "What is a CHT? Is that like a doctor?"

"Well, a CHT is highly trained in the practice of hydrocolonic therapy," the receptionist answered.

"So, they *are* doctors?" I asked.

"Do you mean medical doctors?" she said.

Did I mean medical doctors? Was there another kind? Witch doctors, maybe?

"Well, no, they're not *technically* medical doctors," she confessed.

Not *technically*? What did that mean, exactly? *Yeah, well, I'm not technically a rocket scientist.*

If I was uneasy at first, this revelation did nothing to build my confidence. I was about to pay $120 to let myself be temporarily transformed into a human water balloon, and the person in charge was not *technically* a medical doctor. This was shaping up to be one big leap of faith.

Moments later I emerged from the changing room dressed only in a medical gown (the one common denominator between this place and a real medical facility), walked into the procedure room, and waited for my CHT.

She introduced herself, in a French accent, as Sophie. No older than thirty-five, she was five feet five with fair skin and straight, strawberry blond hair cut just above her shoulders. Beneath her form-flattering, white, floral-patterned sundress, Sophie possessed a petite and well-proportioned frame. Her calves were lean but toned, and her breasts struck the perfect balance between a prepubescent and Dolly Parton. She had a sophisticated, worldly look to her that I found incredibly sexy. A quick glance at her fingers told me she apparently was not married. *Bonjour, Sophie!*

I was reminded of what I had been missing out on all these years. Presumably there were more women like Sophie back in France … probably a lot more. Of course, I couldn't be sure.

Sophie gave me a brief overview of what I could expect during the next hour: basically—I'm paraphrasing here—she was going to slip a hose into my butt, turn on the faucet, fill me with as much liquid as I could tolerate, and then reverse the two-way valve to let my body release all that and more.

Then came the kicker: we were going to repeat this process five or six times—that day. I then laid back and saw the poster they had taped to the ceiling above me. No kidding, it was a cat, barely cling-ing to a branch of a tree. The caption read "Oh shit!"

Exactly.

Out of my peripheral vision, I watched Sophie apply a generous amount of K-Y jelly to the white plastic speculum. The length and girth of the speculum were large enough to be, let's say, attention-getting. It was one thing to have something that size *exit* my body, but quite another, I could only imagine, to have something that size *enter* my body. Was I out of my mind? I looked at the cat on the ceiling. He offered no reassurance. Sadly, there was nothing we could do to help each other.

"I'm going to need you to roll onto your side," Sophie said, "so I can put the speculum in place."

After I rolled myself into position, Sophie bent over, speculum in her latex-gloved hand, and inadvertently gave me a direct view right down the front of her dress, where the one thing I did *not* see was a bra.

Trés bien, Sophie, trés bien! I have *to go to Paris.*
To distract myself from the unpleasantness of what was to come, I let my mind drift into a full-on sexual fantasy with Sophie. My fantasy was building momentum. Simultaneously Sophie was beginning the insertion process. As I wore nothing besides a flimsy gown, there was no possibility my sexy CHT could have failed to notice the hardened physical byproduct that arose from my sordid daydream.

My first reaction was run-of-the-mill embarrassment. That was short lived. Then I was overcome with a mild case of speculum envy. Just how did I measure up to this piece of plastic, anyway? I couldn't get a definite answer to this question; the object of my envy was no longer visible.

Seconds later the worst thought occurred to me. Did Sophie think my erection was from fantasizing about her, or did she think it was a reaction to having this large, lubed object deep inside me? Did she think I might be gay? This *was* San Francisco, after all. I spent the next few minutes trying to figure out how to let her know I was heterosexual.

My preoccupation with clarifying my sexual orientation came to a screeching halt when Sophie threw the switch and unleashed a torrent of liquid into my backside. *Ooh la la!*

What exactly was this liquid, anyway? Sophie told me it was water that had been filtered and temperature-regulated.

Filtered? Temperature-regulated? It sounded remarkably similar to the language used in ads by beer companies to describe their brewing process. For all I knew, I was being filled from a warm keg of Miller Genuine Draft.

How much water would my body accept? She informed me most beginners could tolerate about five minutes of filling. With a little practice, some veterans have been known to endure nine or ten minutes. Competitive by nature, I saw this as a challenge. Why settle for average? But because this was an activity I had *no* interest in practicing or mastering, I had to go for the gold *today*. I'd show those veterans. In my mind, I decided I would settle for nothing less than eight minutes.

"Now, Tim, just try to relax, and breathe through the discomfort," Sophie told me. "You're doing great so far. Just breathe through the pain."

I had grossly underestimated how physically difficult this was going to be. I was in a serious state of discomfort, close to my breaking point. The thought of water balloons being filled to the bursting point was not a particularly helpful visual.

"How long has it been?" I asked.

"Coming up on three minutes," she said.

So much for breaking the record. I'd be lucky to last another thirty seconds. It was easy for me to rationalize abandoning my competitive time goal. Even if I did walk away with the new world record, who was I going to tell? *Hey guys, guess what? Yeah, check this out. I just went eleven full minutes having water pumped into my colon!* Let's face it, what good was winning if I couldn't brag about it? Besides Erin and maybe Steve, I wasn't planning on telling anybody about my colonic, let alone bragging about it.

It was all I could to breathe my way through the four-minute mark before begging Sophie to stop the flooding. She smiled and told me that four minutes wasn't too bad for a beginner. I was humbled—not to mention grotesquely bloated.

Sophie reversed the two-way valve. As quickly as the tide had come in, it made its way out. Relief was now in sight—literally.

I watched in amazement as the clear fluid exited through the narrow tube. It wasn't leaving my body at a leisurely pace; it was being propelled with the force and speed of a Jacuzzi jet. I'd never even had a shower with water pressure this strong. *Forget about calling the fire department. I'm your man. Just point me in the right direction.*

Despite the high-pressure outflow, the releasing process lasted nearly as long as the filling process. After several minutes, I wished the tube were not transparent.

When the waters of the Mississippi River recede after flooding the southern plains, it's not just the water that recedes. The river's pull is so powerful it often carries away tons of soil, sediment, and a fair amount of small furniture, too.

Of all the awkward moments I had experienced since making this appointment, this was by far the most uncomfortable and bizarre. I was lying on my back. Sexy Sophie was massaging my stomach muscles to facilitate the releasing process. Our eyes were fixated on the clear tube. Together we watched as this river carried away what had previously been residing inside me. What possible words could we exchange at a time like this? *So, how 'bout those Niners?*

No, only one word could capture this moment.

Merde!

After five more fill-and-release cycles, my first colonic appointment had almost come to an end. Believe it or not, Sophie said I could expect to sit on the toilet in the changing room for another twenty minutes or so to let my body complete the elimination process. It was a half hour before I was clothed and completely drained.

Out in the reception room, Sophie greeted me with a cup of hot herbal tea. *Merci, Sophie.* She claimed this tea had special healing properties that would help restore balance to my body and my spirit. *Whatever.*

She took a step toward me and gave me a big hug; all patients received an end-of-session hug from their CHT. She held me for four or five seconds. I had begun to believe my sex drive had been flushed from my body along with everything else. It now had been restored. *Merci beaucoup!*

It was five o'clock. *Au revoir, Sophie.*

When I picked up Erin two hours later, I had no idea if the colonic had flushed my digestive tract of all its impurities or not. But surprisingly, I did know confiding in Erin purged a lot of my anxiety and set the stage for a great date. When she wanted to hear every last detail about my wacky adventure, I realized I had underestimated her. She was cool as shit.

It would be hard to imagine a more cathartic day.

Web of Deceit

The narrow hallway stretched on forever. I trudged forward, no longer in a hurry. I turned my eyes down toward the worn beige carpet and away from the harsh glare of the fluorescent overhead lighting. My black, faux-leather computer briefcase, swinging tautly from my left shoulder, felt even heavier than usual. When I reached Room 167, I slid the plastic key into the slit, turned the handle, and let my body collapse into the door.

That's when the guilt really kicked in.

"My rental car won't start," I had explained to my prospect's voice mailbox as I cruised down a remote rural road an hour earlier. Only when I realized I was still twenty minutes away and there were no roadside services in sight had my bowels decided to spring into action, intent on sabotaging my morning.

Even though I had an extra pair of identically matching suit pants in the pocket of my computer bag—I'd recently started buying *two* pairs for each suit precisely because I anticipated these types of worst-case scenarios—I couldn't bring myself to keep the appointment. I had to turn around.

"Dead battery," my message had continued. "I'm going to have to reschedule with you next time I'm in town. I apologize for the inconvenience."

The next time I'm in town. Yeah, right. Like I had *any* intention of coming back. Getting from San Francisco to Tucumcari, New Mexico, a tiny city along I-40 halfway in between Albuquerque and Amarillo, was no easy feat. It took two flights and a couple of hours of driving. It was also not cheap. LPM had spent several thousand dollars for me to travel all this way to cancel a meeting. To my disgust, I'd been doing a lot of this lately.

The drive back to the Comfort Inn gave me plenty of time to beat myself up. Had I forgotten *everything* I'd learned in college? It wasn't like Washington and Lee simply *had* an honor system. The place was *built* on the honor system, with each student swearing to live by a simple code: "I will not lie, cheat, or steal." It was a way of life that I took seriously and subscribed to willingly. It was a standard I'd expected to hold myself to long after graduation. Who had I become?

Back in my hotel room, I accepted that the damage had been done. Since I'd already cleared my schedule for the morning, I figured I might as well put the time to good use by trying to make sure this kind of thing would never happen again. Four more colonic sessions with Sophie hadn't led to any noticeable improvement. It was time for drastic measures. This clean-cut boy next door from the East Coast suburbs decided to try something even more unorthodox than hydrocolonic therapy.

I remembered seeing a research study on the Internet that had made a strong empirical case for treating IBS with hypnosis. Putting aside my reluctance to believe *anything* posted on the Internet, I had a feeling that there might be something to the idea that you could use your thoughts to treat your body.

After all, it was obvious to me the relationship between my mind and my body worked perfectly well in reverse—always in a destructive way. Just as Pavlov's dogs salivated when they heard the bell, the mere *thought* of having an accident triggered an instantaneous physiological reaction that would all but guarantee having the very kind of accident I was trying to avoid. It happened every single time, regardless of how many times I'd already relieved myself. Not only had I always suspected my problem wasn't purely physical, but I also thought that over the years, I might have actually conditioned my body to behave this way.

So now I wondered: could this dynamic also work the other way? Through hypnosis, could I reprogram the haywire communication between my brain and my gut? Could hypnosis return me to the confident person I had been when I graduated from college fourteen years earlier? Intuitively, despite my natural inclination to chalk the whole field up to hocus-pocus, there was something about it that made sense. In an odd way, it seemed like it could work.

Now all I needed to do was find a qualified hypnotist who treated people with IBS. There was no doubt in my mind I would find one near San Francisco. As the alternative medicine capital of the United States, the Bay Area was overflowing with every conceivable kind of unconventional practitioner ... every kind, that was, except for hypnotists trained in treating irritable bowels.

Just as I was losing hope, I scrolled down to the bottom of the search results and read about a guy in England—a certified hypnotherapist—who not only treated people with IBS, he *specialized* in it.

Even though I could think of no better reason to finally get on a plane and make my first trip overseas, it turned out I didn't even have to. In exchange for one hundred U.S. dollars, he promised to send me a set of audio recordings that mirrored his one-on-one sessions. Still somewhat hesitant to fork over a hundred bucks, I poked around his site for a few minutes. Reading through the marketing text, I felt as if he were speaking directly to me and to me alone.

How many times have you stayed indoors in case you needed the toilet?

How many holidays and days out have been cancelled because of IBS?

Do you plan shopping trips with military precision around those shops that have toilets?

This was incredible. There was no way he could have known all this about me unless he'd hired a private investigator to follow me around and place a wiretap on my brain. But that seemed unlikely—I didn't even know the guy. If I had any remaining hesitation about this purchase, it vanished when I read the next line.

How many days have you taken off work because of IBS?

That did it. *What the hell!* It was easy to justify throwing down my credit card, especially when I considered all the money I'd saved as a result of not having been on any dates in over a month.

Despite my being up front with Erin about my unique bathroom challenges, our five-month relationship had recently buckled under the constant friction caused by my rigid insistence on planning ahead and avoiding toiletless settings at all costs. Too many conversations had gone too much like this:

Erin:	"Would you come with me to my friend's wedding shower this weekend?"
Me:	"It depends. Where is it?"
Erin:	"In Berkeley."
Me:	"What time does it start? How many people will be there?"
Erin:	"Around noon. Probably fifty or a hundred people, I guess."
Me:	"Is it at someone's house?"
Erin:	"Yes."
Me:	"How big is the house?"
Erin:	"I don't know. I've never been there. Why would the *size* of the house possibly matter?"
Me:	"It just does. Trust me."
Erin:	"Fine. Look, if you don't *want* to go, then why don't you just come out and say so?"

I was utterly incapable of spontaneity, the very thing that made Erin tick. It wasn't my IBS that had done us in; it was the bickering we couldn't overcome. The most depressing aspect of breaking up with Erin was that she was cooler and more understanding about my condition than I imagined any human being could ever be. This was all the more reason to shell out a few extra bucks for overnight delivery of my hypnosis recordings.

Since I still had some free time on my hands before driving back to the Albuquerque airport, I decided to make one more stop on the Internet—this time for something far more out of character for me than hypnosis.

◆   ◆   ◆

"Nice apartment, especially for a guy," Stacey said, standing in my foyer. "I'm impressed."

"Thanks," I said. "What can I get you to drink? I've got Bud Light, merlot, and Jägermeister."

While I hung her coat in the front closet, she strolled into the living room, apparently opting for the self-guided tour. "I'd love a glass of wine. Thank you."

After I read her Match.com profile, Stacey and I had exchanged e-mails for close to a week. Tonight was the first time we'd met in person. I had to admit I'd gone into our first date with a bad attitude.

Thanks to the first eight women I'd met online, and subsequently treated to dinner and margaritas at Café Marimba, I'd quickly become disillusioned with Internet dating. Putting it as diplomatically as I can, there was an undeniable abundance of women in their late twenties and early thirties marketing themselves—deceptively, in my opinion—with the help of circa-1986 spring-break photos.

But when Stacey walked up to meet me in front of Marimba, she was not at all the woman I had pictured in my mind. Incredibly, compared to the online photo showing this olive-skinned brunette mischievously drinking a giant margarita underneath a palm tree, she looked even more attractive in real life. Somebody who looked better in person than in her ad? My friends would never believe it.

I thought the picture in my profile, taken just a few weeks earlier, was the epitome of truth in advertising. Even Elise agreed my photo and self-descriptive sales pitch were right on target. I wasn't pretending to be someone I wasn't.

True, I'd used a little prudent omission in an effort to put my best foot forward, but *everybody* did that. Nobody advertised their flaws, quirks, or defects up front. Nobody mentioned they were obsessed with getting married by Christmas, or they had been diagnosed as bipolar, or they had been served with multiple restraining orders. But believe me, those people *were* out there.

So, yes, by not mentioning my IBS, I suppose I hadn't exactly laid *all* my cards on the table. That was why people went on dates—so they could get to know another human being and, over time, learn all about the little idiosyncrasies that would make some wince but that would cause the right person to shout out, "Call off the search. I've found my soul mate!"

In hindsight IBS wasn't the only detail I should have omitted from my ad.

I never anticipated that mentioning that I had majored in French would be such a double-edged sword. It was a calculated attempt to make women think I was smart, interesting, and worldly. To that extent, my ploy worked beautifully. This was an easy conversational handle they all grabbed onto.

What I hadn't counted on, however, were the inevitable second-level inquiries. To study the language so exhaustively, but then never visit the country? Well, *that* demanded an explanation. The ensuing line of questioning always carried a disapproving, judgmental tone, usually leaving me on the defensive for the duration of what most often turned out to be a short-lived first, and only, date.

If I were to believe everything I read, then every woman on Match.com was an easygoing, down-to-earth girl next door who felt every bit as comfortable in a T-shirt, jeans, and a baseball cap as she did in a formal black dress at the opera. Also, every woman *loved* international travel (Thailand and Fiji, I'd noticed, were the most frequently cited destinations), lived to try chic new restaurants, and generally thrived on the rush of not knowing what was waiting around the next corner.

Deep down I was hoping to find just *one* woman who was as disingenuous about her need for spontaneity as she was about her appearance. So far, no dice.

Of course, Stacey was no different. Even though we had managed to get through the conversational roadblock about France, I knew we weren't compatible in the long run. It was the same old story.

At work and with women, I felt like a fraud. The great-first-impression thing—my trademark—had become a curse because it set all the wrong expectations. People gave me jobs and set me up with their girlfriends because they thought highly of me. Eventually, I was convinced, they would all see through me. Once the curtain was pulled back, and my secret revealed, then all my good fortune would disappear. At the moment, Stacey had no way of seeing all this, yet I knew it was only a matter of time before she would.

The more I thought about it, the more I questioned the wisdom of focusing so intently on the long run. If my jobs and relationships were ultimately destined for failure anyway, then why shouldn't I enjoy whatever short-term financial or sexual opportunities came my way? Was there any reason, I had wondered to myself over our second pitcher of margaritas, for things not to work out between Stacey and me *tonight*?

When I walked back into the living room with two glasses of wine, Stacey was stretched out along my couch. When I first got into copier sales, Jeff had taught me about this kind of thing. This, he had said, was what was known as a buying signal. And when the customer gives you a buying signal, that's when you shut up, stop selling, and close the deal.

I set the wine glasses on my coffee table, dimmed the lights, and sat down next to her on the couch. Everything was perfect. Nothing left to do except ...

"Why don't you put on some music?" she asked.

Music! How could I have forgotten the music?

Without taking my eyes away from hers, I grabbed the remote for my stereo from my coffee table's lower shelf. After minimal fumbling, my fingers managed to locate both Power and Play in quick succession.

The soft, blue glow from my stereo's lights added the perfect romantic touch to the otherwise dark room. I reached out and put my hand on hers. Aside from the beating of my heart, the only sound was the shuffling start-up noise from my six-disc CD player.

I couldn't remember if we were about to hear Chris Isaak's *Forever Blue* or Neil Diamond's *Greatest Hits*. No matter. At least I'd remembered to take the Jerky Boys out of the rotation.

Our mouths grew closer. I pressed my lips gently against hers. Maybe it was the margaritas, but there was none of the usual awkwardness. As our kiss continued, I felt her warm, soft hand touch the back of my neck. Slowly she pulled me closer, but in an aggressive way. I watched her eyes flicker shut, and then I closed mine. This was no time for talking. Words would only get in the way.

Soft, tender piano notes floated through my speakers and into the room.

Hmmm ... definitely not Neil Diamond.

I let out a low moan as Stacey's hands moved to my back, her fingernails tracing my spine.

Wait ... doesn't sound like Chris Isaak, either.

I wrapped my arms around the back of her neck. Her breathing grew a little heavier.

"Hello. My name is Michael Mahoney."

What? Who the hell is Michael ...

Simultaneously we both opened our eyes, and our kiss came to a momentary standstill. Stacey looked to me for some kind of explanation. Could she see I was just as baffled?

Wait, maybe this is that classical CD my mom sent me. So … this Mahoney guy … I guess he's the conductor or something?

"I'm a clinical hypnotherapist in the United Kingdom," said a man with a mellow, soothing British accent.

No! No! No! No! No! No!

I struggled to disentangle my arms from Stacey's neck. Our passion ground to a screeching halt. Scrambling for the remote, I knocked it off the coffee table. Exactly where it landed, I wasn't sure. I thrust my hand down toward the floor, groping the sisal rug for any signs of the slippery piece of plastic.

OK, don't lose your cool. So far all she knows is that you've got a hypnosis CD. She has no idea what it's for. You can still recover … but you have to find that remote before this guy says anything else.

Hooking my forearm underneath the couch in a way that made me think I might just have a future as a circus contortionist, I found the elusive remote. Still, it was hard to get a firm grip on the little bastard. I reached farther, this time adding a twisting motion to my wrist. With two fingers now on top of the object, all I had to do was drag it toward—

"The last twelve years have been spent treating irritable bowel syndrome."

That's it. Game over. I am toast!

With the remote control now finally in my grasp, I retracted my arm from underneath the sofa and jammed my thumb into the power button. Then, turning to hide my face, I reached for my glass of wine and took a big, long gulp.

"I don't know about you, but I could use a refill." I stood up and walked toward the kitchen.

No question about it: the date was officially over. But before we parted ways, there still remained the awkward process of exchanging insincere pleasantries while pretending that what had just happened hadn't, in fact, just happened. I didn't know what to say.

Stacey did.

"It's getting late. I really should go." She pulled out her cell phone. "Yes, hello, I need a cab, please. I'm on Broderick Street … in the

Marina ... Yes, I *am* ready now. Thank you." She started walking toward to the front door.

"Don't you want to wait here until the cab comes?" I asked.

"No, that's sweet of you. The guy said they'd send a car right over. Thank you for a nice night."

I didn't want to say another word, but I felt oddly compelled. "I'll give you a call. Maybe we can see each other again?" *How pathetic.*

"Yeah, sure. That would be nice," she said, scurrying down the hall toward the staircase. She couldn't get gone fast enough.

I looked down at my watch. It was only eleven o'clock. The last thing I wanted to do was spend the rest of the night alone. I was feeling a little needy ... desperate for companionship.

I lay back down on the couch, pulled a blanket over myself, and hit Play.

Listening to the rhythm of his calm, soothing voice felt like being on a mild sedative. Even though I was perfectly aware of my surroundings, it was as if I'd been transformed into a limp, drowsy sack of potatoes that had, at least temporarily, no capacity whatsoever to worry.

In fact, I was in such a peaceful state that I felt like I was going to fall asleep before he was finished talking to me. But he insisted this was perfectly fine because my subconscious was taking in his every word. Only fifteen minutes into the half-hour recording, I couldn't fight it off anymore. I was out for the night.

◆　　　◆　　　◆

"Who are you going to bring?"

"Well, Mom," I said, "I'm not planning on bringing anybody."

For a few long seconds, I was sure the line had gone dead.

"Hello?"

"You're going to show up at your brother's wedding without a date?"

"At the moment, yeah, it's kind of looking that way."

"Tim, I'm honestly worried about you," my mom said in a tone suggesting that what she honestly felt was sorry for me. "You're thirty-six and still single. The problem is that you're only going to get *more* rigid and set in your ways than you already are."

This was her way of encouraging me?

"If you wait too long," she said, "nobody's going to want to marry you. Personally, I think you have a fear of commitment."

Fear of commitment. She threw this tired cliché my way as if this were a new concept to me, as if hundreds of women hadn't already leveled this charge at me over the years. God knew there were tons of things I feared. Commitment, however, was not one of them.

In fact, if I wasn't looking for a commitment, I never would have gone back to Match.com to throw out some more feelers. My mom was wrong. She didn't understand.

After the misstep with Stacey, I spent hour after hour combing through hundreds of profiles, looking for my ideal woman. I would know instantly when I found her. My princess would be the rare catch who flew underneath everyone else's radar—a woman so comfortable in her own skin that her profile would read something very close to this:

My ideal date:

Stay in, order a pizza, and rent a classic movie like Caddyshack *or* Airplane!

My turn-ons:

I'm a sucker for a logical, analytical man who is meticulous about planning everything in advance. My prince will also be the man who isn't afraid to admit his insecurities. Extra points if he also has the good sense to avoid traveling during rush hour.

My turn-offs:

I'd rather die than spend a long, stuffy evening at the opera or the symphony. I cringe at the thought of taking long trips to interesting places where I've never been before.

Sadly, despite my wishful thinking, I failed to uncover my home-body in the haystack. That didn't mean she wasn't out there. It just meant that she, along with everybody else, was full of crap, pretending to be somebody she wasn't. Until I figured out this IBS thing, it was futile, demoralizing, and also really expensive to keep pursuing these online Indiana Jones types.

I didn't tell my mom, but taking a self-imposed break from Match.com hadn't prevented me from making what I considered to be a serious commitment to somebody else.

We'd only had four dates. Yet each morning, I woke up and found myself looking forward to the time we were going to spend together. At the office and at the gym, the hours crawled by as I longed for the night to roll around.

Maybe it's because they're at once so uncertain and so full of promise, but new relationships always invigorate me. I didn't want to jinx myself, but there was something about this one that just felt right to me.

I'd been with some aggressive people before, but nobody had ever gotten me to agree to a set of formalized ground rules. I was hesitant, but eventually agreed to two such rules: First, we would spend time together every day. Second, neither of us would walk away before one hundred days had passed. I couldn't imagine going along with such a rigorous plan with anybody else, but there was something special about this Michael Mahoney guy.

I walked in from the gym around six thirty, filled with anticipation. After taking a moment to watch the setting sun dip below the Golden Gate Bridge, I lowered my blinds, turned off the living room lights, and reclined on my couch.

I had the CD already queued up.

The session began with the reminder that these recordings were for people who had been diagnosed by their doctors with irritable bowel syndrome, followed by a warning to resist the temptation to self-diagnose. *Too late.*

As soon as I heard, "I want you to take three long, deep breaths," I could feel my body wilt. By my third breath, I was halfway to la-la land. A few more words, and I'd be all the way there.

"You were not born with IBS. Somewhere in your history, you have a memory of living life without IBS."

That's true. I can almost remember what my life used to be like, way back when.

"Each thought about IBS has an effect on your body. Repeated thoughts, every day, make IBS more a part of you. Hypnosis will help you break this cycle."

This guy really understands me.

"Subconscious thoughts make things worse, too. What-if thoughts can trigger your symptoms … just the thought of it. Each time you have one of these thoughts, you are reinforcing the thought pattern and the grooves that keep IBS with you. We need to change the way we think to ourselves about IBS."

Michael, I wouldn't be here if I wasn't willing to try. I just hope you're right.

I didn't remember anything he said after this because, once again, I passed out. I swear, there was something magical about that guy's voice.

When I woke up, I turned my phone back on. I had a message from my brother.

"Hey, Tim. It's Fred. I just wanted to get back to you with answers to *all* of your questions about the wedding. Melissa and I are getting married at twelve noon on May 18. That's a Saturday. The name of the church is Saint Margaret Mary. It's in Omaha and about a fifteen-minute drive from my apartment. The reception will start at five o'clock … that's also on Saturday. We're expecting 350 guests. It's going to be a Catholic Mass, so it will probably only last for about an hour … you know, give or take. You'll need to wear a tuxedo."

I grabbed a pen to jot down all the details, which were only getting more terrifying as his message rambled on. He hadn't even gotten to the good stuff yet.

"As far as your best-man duties are concerned ..."

Fred had caught me off guard with this request a few weeks earlier. How could I possibly say no to my brother? This was one of the most important days of his life, and I wanted to be there for him.

"Yes, of course I'll be your best man," I'd said. "I'm honored." It was probably a good thing I'd said yes before I knew exactly what my role would entail.

"... all you have to do at the church is stand next to me during the ceremony and hold on to the rings. Then later on, at the reception, you stand up on the stage and entertain everybody with a toast. Nothing to it. OK, gotta run. Later, dude."

One hour at the altar? Entertain 350 people with a toast? I can't do this. There's no way.

Unfortunately this wasn't a sales call that I could cancel. There was no way I could back out of this commitment. I couldn't quit the family, either. For better or for worse, I was locked in.

Michael Mahoney was my best hope. The wedding was exactly eighty-five days away. If I stayed on track, I'd be done with my hypnosis CDs in eighty-three.

Tying the Knot

"Can I get a margarita on the rocks, please?" I said. "With an extra shot of tequila, if you don't mind."

"Hi, Tim. I'm Doris Schumacher. I'm a friend of Melissa's parents. I just wanted to say I enjoyed your toast. It was funny, but also very touching. I'm sure it meant a lot to your brother."

"Thank you," I said, slugging down my margarita. "That's very nice of you to say."

"Now I hope you'll pardon me for being so direct … but did I hear you're *single*?"

"Yes," I said, motioning to the bartender for a quick refill. "That's correct."

"Again, I hope you'll forgive me, but how can that be?"

"Excuse me?" I said, nearly coughing up my cocktail.

"I mean why hasn't an eligible bachelor like you been snatched off the market yet?"

I reached for my second margarita, took another long sip, and reflected on how my day had unfolded.

◆　　　◆　　　◆

Less than an hour before I had to be at the church, I picked up the phone and called my stepfather. If anybody could help me out of my predicament, John could.

"What's the problem?" my stepfather asked.

"It's my bow tie," I said. "It's not cooperating."

185

"What do you mean, not cooperating?"

"I mean I can't figure out how to tie the damned thing."

"Tim, it can't be that tricky. There's only one way to tie a bow tie."

It was time to swallow my pride. "Well, that's the problem. I've never owned a real bow tie before, so I never learned how to tie one."

John was a die-hard holdout of a bygone formal era, the kind of guy who still bitterly resented the fact that people didn't put on their Sunday best before stepping onto a plane. Predictably, he was incredulous. "How can anybody *not* know how to tie a bow tie? What is it about this generation? I couldn't have been four years old when my father sat me down and showed me ..."

Yeah, that was what I needed: a lecture. I should have just bought the clip-on when I'd bought my first tuxedo a month earlier. But no, that would have been too easy. I had to be a big shot, a show-off. *Look at me. I tied it all by myself!* I had to add another layer of complexity and uncertainty to this morning's mix.

It's not as if I hadn't spent the previous two months dwelling on the challenges of fulfilling my best-man duties. It's not as if I hadn't expected Fred's wedding to be the most stressful, uncomfortable day of my life. Somehow I just never anticipated how difficult it would be to twist and coax a foot-long strip of slippery black silk into the proper shape.

Three weeks before leaving for Omaha, even though I'd made quite a bit of progress, I'd begun to prepare for the possibility that my hypnosis CDs might not render me 100 percent symptom-free in time for my brother's big day. In fairness, Michael Mahoney had specifically warned against expecting such speedy results, but because I was desperate, I chose to ignore the warning. Because I simply could not afford to let my bowels ruin Fred and Melissa's wedding, I decided to map out a foolproof contingency plan.

An intricate operation requiring a vast arsenal of precision supplies, the plan would force me to draw upon every last bit of wisdom I'd accumulated from more than a decade of hard-fought trial and error. It was the kind of plan that, without the correct sequence and exacting timing, didn't stand a chance. The logistics may have been elaborate, but the concept was simple: I was going to throw the kitchen sink at the problem.

The day had gotten off to a good start, albeit an early one at 6:00 AM, when room service delivered a couple of scrambled eggs and one large pot of black coffee. It didn't take long for me to put a check in the box next to Phase I (avalanche blasting). Right on schedule.

It was when I walked over to my suitcase to get Phase II under way that things started to go sideways. I searched my suitcase inside and out, tearing open every compartment. I yanked open all the dresser drawers and searched the closet floor. I even spilled the contents of my dob kit onto the counter. Nothing. I had done the unthinkable. I had left my enema in San Francisco. This was a critical blunder. *Idiot!*

Maybe it was a sign. Maybe it was God's way of saying, "Tim, didn't you already learn your lesson with these things?"

Of course, I was desperate, but I figured as long as I used the enema three or four hours before getting to the church, then I'd have plenty of lead time to let the aftershocks run their course. And besides, this time around, once the enema worked its magic, Phase III called for a supersized Imodium chaser to slow things down again. I had dubbed this experimental combo aspect of the plan the Drain-then-Seal technique.

I don't think I'd ever been so glad to be single. Intimate moments like this were best left unshared. I could only imagine how my morning would have gone if I had listened to my mother and brought along a date.

With no real slack in the schedule, my frantic scouring of downtown Omaha, on foot, in search of a pharmacy open at seven thirty in the morning almost jeopardized the whole plan. By the time I found one and ran back to my room at the Embassy Suites, it was almost eight thirty. Precious time had been lost. I was now cutting it dangerously close, but went ahead with my forced purging anyway. As it had several years earlier, the enema sent me racing to the toilet within minutes with a *strong* need to evacuate.

Two hours later, following a series of violent aftershocks that further gutted my insides, I declared Phase II complete and moved ahead to Phase III by popping a double dose of maximum-strength Imodium to initiate the sealing process.

Now I had a little time to tie up some other essential loose ends, like showering, shaving, and ironing my tuxedo shirt. By eleven o'clock, I was ready for Phase IV—the final touch. I closed the curtains, turned off the lights, and stretched out on the bed to let myself be hypnotized for the hundredth time in as many days.

Once again Michael Mahoney's voice worked its magic. Within seconds my eyelids grew heavy, and all my muscles fell limp. As I plunged into that familiar state of blissful unconsciousness, all my tension, physical and mental, slipped away. I was so relaxed that I was no longer sure if I even had a digestive tract—the ultimate sensation.

If only I could capture this state and call it up on demand, then all my problems would be solved. Wouldn't it be amazing, I fantasized, if instead of panic and instantaneous diarrhea, my body's automatic reaction to anxious situations was this wonderful, near-catatonic calmness produced so easily by these recordings?

Then, as always, I fell asleep—a deep, deep, deep sleep. There was no sense fighting it; at the end of the thirty-minute session Michael always roused me gently back to consciousness by counting backward from ten to one.

Until I heard him whisper "three … two … one … now open your eyes and be fully awake," my only responsibility was to have no responsibility whatsoever. Heaven.

But on the one day I needed it the most, I never heard the wake-up count. I had slept right through it. By the time I woke up, I was relaxed, all right—a feeling that was jarringly replaced by sheer panic when I looked over at the clock and saw how long I'd slept. I was way behind schedule. I scrambled to throw on my tuxedo and my shoes. Then, of course, there was the matter of the bow tie.

Back in San Francisco, Leon, the salesman at the Hound, had walked me through it step-by-step. He even encouraged me to practice on one of the store's mannequins before I left. "No thanks, Leon, it looks pretty straightforward. I think I got it." But for the life of me, here at the Embassy Suites in downtown Omaha, I could *not* get it.

Curiously, despite the spastic jabs of his banana-sized, arthritic fingers, neither could John. After a dozen failed attempts, he finally coerced the silk strip into holding what he assured me was a perfectly acceptable-looking knot.

"There you go," my stepfather said. "It's not my best work, but it will certainly do the trick."

OK, crisis averted. Now let go of the stress, and try to relax again. Everything's going to be just fine. That's it. Take three long, deep breaths. Exhale fully after each one, and feel the tension slip away. That's it. That's it.

Just then somebody pounded on the door.

It was my mom—the wonderful woman whose greatest shortcoming, in my loving opinion, was that she'd spent her life elevating the practice of being frantically late to an art form. She looked as stressed as I'd ever seen her.

"Tim and John, come on. We've *got* to get on the shuttle," my mom shouted in a tone that unnecessarily overstated the direness of the situation. "*Everybody's* already on it. Let's *go!*"

John, a patient man who had the good sense to pick his battles carefully, followed my mom's orders, while I chose to brush them aside. I'd always found my mom's stress to be contagious, so putting maximum physical distance between the two of us was essential to any remaining shot I had of returning to some semblance of my euphoric, posthypnotic state.

"Go ahead," I said to my mom, as calmly as I could manage. "I'll take the next shuttle."

"There is no *next* one, Tim. This is it!"

"Don't worry," I said. "I know where the church is. I'll get there. Just ... go ... ahead."

"Tim, I'm telling you. Come on. That makes no sense. Let's just walk outside and get on the bus. You can't be late. We have to be there for the pictures. The photographer's waiting."

Unlike an hour earlier, I was now all too aware that I had a digestive tract. Now I really had to use the bathroom again. Where was Michael Mahoney when I needed him?

"Mom! Drop it, OK? I already told you that I will meet you there!"

"John, please talk some sense into him. He *can't* miss the shuttle. *Tell* him." She was now bordering on hysteria. Tears, I knew from experience, would soon follow.

After emerging from my room and what I prayed would be my last toilet trip of the day, I waited in the lobby until I saw the shuttle bus leave for the church. When the coast was clear, I went to the bathroom one more time. Then I stepped outside and into a cab.

I knew from going to the rehearsal there were plenty of places to stop along the way if I had to, but there was no way I was going to risk asking a bus packed with wedding guests to pull over during a short fifteen-minute drive so the best man could make an emergency pit stop. After all, these people were going to be my audience for my big toast at the reception. The last thing I needed was an already-hostile crowd.

When my cab pulled up to the church, the wedding party was already gathered outside. Chatting into her cell phone and rummaging through her camera bag, the photographer looked like she wasn't quite ready to start shooting. I figured I could grab at least two minutes of toilet time inside.

I walked over to Fred, who looked sharp and handsome in his blue air force formal wear. Next to him stood fifteen of his air force buddies decked out in similarly crisp and creased fashion, wearing bow ties whose knots looked so perfect there was no way they could have been tied by human hands.

"Fred, I'm going to duck inside for a minute, and then I'll be right out."

Fred stared at me, horrified.

"What, not enough time?" I asked.

"No, that's not the problem," he said.

"What *is* the problem?"

He stared for a few more seconds before blurting out, "Dude, what the *fuck* is up with your tie?"

"What do you mean? John tied it. What's wrong with it?"

He grabbed me by the arm and pulled me into the parking lot. My reflection, seen in the window of a Buick Cutlass, told the tale.

"I'm no expert, but I don't think it's supposed to look like *that*. You've got to fix it."

The photographer, still holding her phone to her ear, walked by, gave me a critical once-over, and nodded in emphatic agreement.

Tied around my neck was what could only be described as a set of mutant Mickey Mouse ears from Disney World. They were so absurdly deformed and lopsided that the right ear dwarfed the size of the left ear by a factor of ten. In any other setting, my appearance would have been hilarious.

I called John, the self-proclaimed expert who had bragged he could tie a bow tie in his sleep, back over to make things right. His massive fingers came at me again, waving in front of my face like giant octopus tentacles. Try as he might, he just couldn't get the knot to look as it should. But worst of all, every time-consuming attempt robbed me of valuable toilet time.

"There's something wrong with this tie," John said. "Where did you buy this thing?"

A small crowd of wedding guests had now gathered to watch the dramatic spectacle play out.

"What does it matter where I bought it?" I said. "It's a perfectly good tie. Why can't you just tie it?"

When it became apparent the chances of a successful outcome were shrinking with each passing minute, Gianfranco, my sister's fiancé and a former Marine, raced down to the formal-wear shop to see if he could save the wedding by procuring a $15, clip-on bow tie.

Meanwhile John's fumbling fingers continued to fly in front of my face. As if witnessing a woefully inept magician attempting to saw a volunteer from the audience in half, the now-nervous onlookers were enthralled. Actually, at the time, being sawed in two sounded pretty good. At least then my lower half could run inside and use the toilet.

◆   ◆   ◆

The organ music was my cue. With a final flush, I bolted from the men's room in the church basement. For the next hour, this sanctuary would be off-limits to me just when I would need it the most.

I ran into my brother in the hallway. "This is serious, Tim," Fred said, his voice cracking. "I'm scared, man. Any words of wisdom?"

He was asking *me* for advice? I'd been so wrapped up in my own blanket of fear I hadn't considered what he might be going through. He was about to take the most monumental step of his life. All I had to do was to stand next to him for an hour and, when the time came, reach into my pocket and hand him the two wedding bands.

The only words I could offer were the ones I'd been repeating to myself since my final flush.

"Do you remember *The Right Stuff*?" I asked.

"Yeah."

"You know when Alan Shepard is sitting in his capsule waiting for liftoff?"

"Kind of," Fred said, confused.

"Anyway, while the whole world is watching, waiting for this courageous, superhuman pilot to blast off into orbit and make history, Shepard says to himself, 'Oh dear God, please don't let me fuck up.'"

Fred had no idea what I was talking about. What did this have to do with anything?

I grabbed him by the shoulders and looked him in the eye. "What I'm saying is that even though you feel scared, you're still doing the right thing."

I followed him from the basement up into the church, trying to make myself believe the words I'd just uttered.

As the best man, I would escort the maid of honor down the aisle, but that wasn't going to happen right away. As the final pairing, Ann and I were currently number six in line for departure.

I passed the time by looking back at the stairs leading to the basement. *You don't have time to go again. You can't risk it. But if you were really quick …*

Five slow pairings later, I locked arms with Ann and put my right foot in front of my left.

Why is everybody looking at us?

Hundreds of eyeballs. Such scrutiny.

Don't they have anything better to do?

It didn't seem to matter that I'd eaten almost nothing in the previous forty-eight hours, or that I'd undergone one hundred consecutive hypnosis sessions, or that I'd gone to greater lengths than anybody in history to empty his digestive tract. No, incredibly, at this moment, none of this seemed to matter. My body was telling me there was still more … not a lot more, but more nonetheless. I could feel the spasms running down the length of my colon.

Looking to my left, I saw only strangers staring as we marched past.

Who are these people? Do I look as scared as I am? Are they judging me? Probably.

I turned to my right, where at least I could see people I knew: uncles, aunts, cousins, nieces, nephews, and my grandfather, too. Their smiles should have comforted me, but they didn't. They were proud of me for the role I was playing in my brother's shining moment. Would they still be proud if I had a mishap here in front of everybody? More spasms pulsed through the length of my midsection.

Ann and I reached the front row and went our separate ways. Everybody turned around again. My younger brother began his march to the altar, taking his last steps as a single man. He'd always been the fearless one in the family. And even though he looked calm, cool, and confident as he strode toward the first day of the rest of his committed life, I knew what was going through his mind.

When Fred reached the altar, and all the supporting players were in place, "Here Comes the Bride" bellowed from the organ and reverberated through the cavernous cathedral. All eyes turned toward the back of the church. It was the bride's turn to bask in the limelight.

As she strode gracefully past the pews, I watched a smile wash across my brother's face. The nearer Melissa walked, the more relaxed and happy Fred appeared.

That made one of us. For perhaps the first time in recorded history, the best man was more petrified than the groom.

With each step Melissa took, another full row of family, friends, and complete strangers turned to look once again toward the front of the church—to look once again toward me. The closer my future sister-in-law got, the more belligerent my bowels became. But with Melissa approaching the first row, it was way too late for me to go anywhere. Like my younger brother, I was now committed.

While a black tuxedo would help conceal any embarrassing stains, it didn't help that as the only civilian among the groomsmen, I was the only one *not* wearing air force blue. As the only man dressed in black and white, I wouldn't be too difficult to identify as the skunk at this picnic.

Sneaking a glance at my watch, I saw that I still had fifty minutes to endure. *Oh dear God, please don't let me fuck up.*

I couldn't possibly imagine how much more pressure must come along with being the groom. Forget about the ceremony. What about the honeymoon? I still hadn't set foot outside the continental United States. Where would I possibly find a woman willing to follow up our nuptials with a summer road trip along I-40 so we could take in the Grand Canyon? Every couple I'd ever known went *at least* as far as Europe … and lately, that was even becoming frowned upon as too ho-hum.

When the time came for Fred and Melissa to exchange their vows, I fantasized about someday doing the same. *Do you, Bowels, promise to love and support this man, to obey him, in good times and bad, for better or worse, in sickness and in health, until death do you part?*

Until that day came along, my mom was just going to have to accept the fact that being Fred's best man was as close as I was going to get to getting married.

"I now pronounce you husband and wife," said the priest. "You may kiss the bride."

Amen. I'd made it through the Mass.

◆   ◆   ◆

Why wasn't I married yet? I could forgive Doris Schumacher for asking the question. After all, she'd only seen me for the ten minutes I was onstage with the microphone, in all my glory.

Ironically, after getting through the first minute or so, I'd never felt so confident in my entire life. I was on center stage, and I was making a roomful of people laugh and cheer. I was in the zone and didn't even *think* about going to the bathroom.

If the compliments that followed were sincere, then I had successfully delivered one of the finest, most entertaining best-man toasts of all time. Complete strangers came up to me with comments like, "Great job! You nailed it!" My brother's pilot buddies, rendered less articulate by the open bar, were just as effusive with their praise: "Awesome, dude! Totally awesome!"

But most important, Fred and Melissa loved it. I've never seen my brother laugh and smile so much.

Why wasn't I married yet?

I shot her a grin and delivered my standard sarcastic quip. "Just lucky, I guess." I threw in a chuckle and a wink to let her know I was just joking around.

"Very funny," she said. "But I'm not buying it."

Doris was waiting for a more serious answer. She'd have to wait a few more seconds.

I was still relishing the moment, still sky-high from the applause, the laughter, and the praise. I wasn't just the man; for those unforgettable ten minutes, I was truly the *best* man.

At that moment, standing at the bar with my margarita and the intoxicating feeling of absolute invincibility, I believed I could do *anything*—including someday tying my own knot.

"That's a good question, Doris," I said. "Honestly, I couldn't begin to tell you why."

Brave New World

"Good evening, Mr. Phelan. Would you care for a glass of champagne?"

"Do you happen to have any Jägermeister?"

"Jägermeister? No, I'm afraid not."

"Well, then I suppose champagne will be fine, thank you."

I reached for the glass and stared out the window. A pivotal moment if there ever was one. Now that it was finally happening, it was surreal. No matter what happened next, the important thing was that I was here. I was doing it. Nobody could take that away from me.

My buddy Drew had called two months earlier with the invitation. Would I be interested in joining him and six other guys for a week-long golf vacation in Ireland? Listening to him describe the camaraderie and the historic courses we would play, I surprised myself by not cutting to the chase and politely saying, "Damn, I wish I could go, but August just doesn't work for me."

Instead I suppressed all my instincts and actually mulled it over.

Drew had unknowingly timed his call perfectly. Part of me—the part that had been unwillingly celibate for way too many months—was growing increasingly hostile. It pissed me off that my lack of international travel had become something of a liability in the dating arena. I felt like I had something to prove to the women of San Francisco … and more important, to myself.

Another part of me was still basking in the confidence of having gotten through Fred's wedding unscathed. Never mind the absurd lengths I'd resorted to. Ultimately I *had* done it. Ever since I got back from

Omaha, I'd been daydreaming about what other once-unimaginable feats might now be within my reach.

Drew kept talking. I kept listening.

It helped that I already knew four of the other seven golfers. Still, seven days of driving all around Ireland sounded ambitious—never mind the transatlantic flight itself. God knew I wanted to go. Was this really something I could pull off?

Inspiration can come from the strangest of places. I started thinking about Bowie.

From that summer day in 1982 when my sister, Lisa, brought this mangy, black-and-white mutt home from the pound, Bowie (named for singer David Bowie, who purportedly also has two different-colored eyes) was a restless dog. It wasn't long before my parents installed one of those Invisible Fences.

For weeks we watched and winced as Bowie, who continually strayed too close to the edge of our backyard, recoiled from one electrical shock to his neck after another. The poor dog was in obvious pain, but this negative reinforcement, we were told, would teach Bowie to live within his boundaries and keep him from running away and getting into trouble. "It's for his own good," my parents had explained.

Bowie, it seemed, did not agree.

Maybe he'd hated living with us for those few months. Maybe he had dreamed of a better life with bigger pastures and more squirrels to chase. Who knew? Whatever his motivation, one day Bowie put his fear aside. In a desperate dash for freedom, knowing full well how painful that jolt of electricity would be, he charged right through his Invisible Fence.

That dog had guts.

I'd often thought about my own Invisible Fence. Whenever I approached the edges of my comfort zone, a major shock from my bowels always reminded me exactly where my boundaries were. They knew all too well when I got close to leaving the "safe" areas where toilet locations were known and unfettered access was assured. There was a whole world just waiting for me, calling me, and I'd been too scared to leave my backyard.

That was it. Enough was enough.

Like Bowie, I decided this was no way to live. I'd spent my whole adult life missing out. Now it was time to catch up. What fate awaited me on the other side of my fence? There was only one way to find out.

In an uncharacteristically impulsive move that didn't score me any points with my boss, Paul, I'd decided to use up my full two weeks of vacation time in one fell swoop. If I was going to leave my backyard, I sure as hell wanted to make the most of it.

"Welcome aboard, ladies and gentlemen. I'm Captain Cooper, and it's our pleasure to have you with us tonight. We are anticipating a very short flight of nine hours and thirty-one minutes as we make our way from San Francisco to London's Heathrow airport."

Nine hours and thirty-one minutes. A very short flight?

With an attention-getting nudge, the massive Boeing 777 pushed back from the gate. There was no turning back. We were on our way. For the first time in years, I was more proud than I was scared.

I raised my champagne glass and quietly toasted myself. "Well, it's about time. Thirty-six years old and finally taking your first trip to Europe. Better late than never. Nice job."

"Flight attendants, please prepare for takeoff."

At the end of the runway, the powerful twin engines roared to life. The seat trays and overhead bins vibrated.

For business trips, I'd been at this very spot, poised for takeoff on runway 01 Right, in massive jets like this, more times than I could count. The feeling was so familiar, but also so brand-new. Nobody had ordered me to be there. This was *my* decision. *My* free will.

And this wasn't a business trip. This plane was not going to land in San Diego or Denver or even New York. I was headed for a *new* world, one that I'd been beginning to think I might never see.

All I knew for certain was that my passport was only nine and a half hours away from being stamped for the very first time. Beyond that, however, I didn't have a clue as to what I was in for. Just like Bowie.

For the record, I should mention that while Bowie's courage was never in question, his fate remained a mystery. I liked to think he was still out there somewhere, chasing squirrels, terrorizing chickens, and living the good life. But it was just as likely he met his fate underneath the tires of a speeding BMW or Range Rover along Riversville Road. Once he took off, we never saw him again.

◆   ◆   ◆

The itinerary was a bold one, even for this group of die-hard golf fanatics.

Into a mere seven days, we would cram thirteen rounds of golf. Exhausting as that sounded, the more time spent on the golf course, the better. I'd never encountered a course where, in a pinch, I couldn't find some privacy to relieve myself. Likewise, I was confident all our hotels and inns would have ample facilities.

What worried me most, aside from the *very short* flight from San Francisco, was the day-to-day driving. Beginning on the eastern shore in Dublin and traveling clockwise around the country until we reached Shannon on the island's west coast, we would trace Ireland's southern coastline and play all of the country's storied links courses.

Some days we would only be on the bus for ten minutes. Other days called for two- or three-hour road trips. There were only eight of us, so we didn't spring for a full-sized coach—the kind that might have an onboard lavatory in the back.

At the end of August, squeezing in two rounds of golf before the sun went down was challenging. Since we often had to be on the bus before sunrise, I didn't have time for the hugely successful, but time-consuming, Drain-then-Seal technique I'd unveiled in Omaha and deployed again prior to the flight over to Europe.

My best strategy was to set my alarm for two hours earlier than everybody else, usually around 4:30, and slip down to the dining room. My hope was that eating the morning staple known as the full Irish breakfast (scrambled eggs, blood sausage, toast, and the harsh, raw-tasting, hot beverage that they pronounced "coffee") would render me mostly empty. It was an imperfect plan at best, and most mornings I had no choice but to board the bus with more anxiety than peace of mind.

Because I'd never breathed a word about my irritable bowels to any of these guys, not even Drew (another former co-worker from my days at Robertson Stephens), they were oblivious to the fact that they were traveling with a ticking time bomb.

On our third morning, we had a three-hour ride from Waterville to Ballybunion. It was only seven o'clock, but the boys were already in full swing in the back of the coach. Adam and Michael were getting a little worked up.

"Hey, Tim, how you doin' up there?" Adam shouted.

Michael, as usual, was more ornery. "Damn it, Phelan, get your ass back here and drink with us, would you?"

No matter how short or long the trip, the guys reflexively retreated to the back row, where they converted the long table into a casino on wheels. Morning, noon, or night, Guinness cans were drained, Marlboros were inhaled, and games like Liar's Poker and Mexican Dice were played for high stakes. Every two years, for the last decade, such had been the tradition with this group.

"I'll come back in a while," I said, citing what I thought might pass for a plausible pretense for riding up front and chatting with our driver, Ger (pronounced "Jair"). "I'm learning all about Ireland."

Ger looked over and said, "Don't let me stop ya from joining the hooley. Go on ahead back thar if ya like."

"No, that's OK," I said. "This is more interesting to me."

Realizing I couldn't pull the bus over for an emergency pit stop, I thought it was prudent to sit next to, and befriend, the one man who could. So far I hadn't been responsible for any unscheduled stops. In a nice twist of fate, the more Guinness cans my traveling companions emptied back in the casino, the more pit stops they needed.

On this morning, driving from Waterville to Ballybunion, I had something bigger than pit stops to worry about. As clearly the worst golfer of the bunch, I was a little intimidated about who my playing partner was today.

I was one of two trip rookies who had been invited when two of the party faithful had opted to pass on this year's excursion. The other first-timer was Bill Monahan. I'd never met him before. I'd only heard about him.

Tall and serious-looking, this blond-haired man, known simply as Bam, was something of a god on this trip. There were respectable golfers on the bus with handicaps of seven or eight, and there were a few really solid golfers who boasted handicaps of three or four.

Then there was Bam.

With a dozen or so tournament wins under his belt, he blew all these guys out of the water. And they knew it. He was the quiet type, a man of few words. Nothing seemed to rattle him. This guy was stoic.

◆   ◆   ◆

Bam's ball sailed off the tee box. At first it looked beautiful. Perfect trajectory. Right on line.

And then it just kept going.

And going. And going.

Flying a good thirty yards past the green, it landed in the thick gorse on the hillside … and literally disappeared.

After a shot like that, winning our match against the Rodgers brothers, Michael and Patrick, would be pretty much out of the question. While I was disappointed, my playing partner had a slightly different take.

Momentarily shedding his image as a man of few words, Bam was livid.

He slammed his four iron into the soggy, rain-soaked grass. "*Motherfucker!* You stupid son of a bitch!" His face turned purple.

This was a meltdown of McEnroe proportions. "What is *wrong* with you? God *damn* it!"

Our caddy, Teddy, was a slim, crusty man who claimed to be in his forties but looked like he was in his early sixties. He had a weathered red face and, at most, a handful of teeth, all scattered randomly, and at various angles, throughout his mouth. Like just about every other caddy we would meet in Ireland, Teddy reeked of both alcohol and tobacco.

Taking a shot of whiskey from his flask and another drag from his cigarette, Teddy waited for Bam to simmer down. Then he walked over, gently wrapped his arm around Bam's shoulder, and tried to help him come to terms with what had just happened.

"So you hit a bad shot," Teddy said. "Tell me, what the fuck can you do about it now?"

Bam was stunned. "What are you saying?"

Teddy took another swig from the flask. "What I'm sayin' is that it doesn't matter how fine a golfer ya are. Everybody hits bad shots. *Everybody.* They're part of the game." Another long drag from his cigarette. "So, when you hit a piece of rubbish like the one you just hit, there are only two things to do."

"What's that?" Bam asked.

Teddy hoisted our bags onto his shoulders. "Forget about your *last* shot."

Bam nodded.

"And then go hit your *next* shot."

As we marched toward the green, the weather turned on us again for the fifth time in fourteen holes. It was a typical day of golf in Ireland. The sun disappeared. The raindrops, propelled horizontally through the air by forty-mile-per-hour wind gusts, ripped into us like bullets. Making matters worse, my ball, while fifty or sixty yards short of Bam's monster shot, also landed in the thick gorse.

Yet none of that fazed me. I was digesting what I'd just heard back on the tee box. *Everybody hits bad shots ... part of the game ... forget about it ... hit your next shot.*

As someone who had only been playing golf for six years, I knew all about bad shots. Every round I'd ever played was littered with them. In the early days, I'd routinely shanked, whiffed, topped, or just plain *lost* 60 percent of the golf balls I swung at. To put it mildly, I sucked.

Yet, inexplicably, I never let the fact that I'd hit so many awful shots (plenty of them were downright embarrassing) keep me from finishing a round or coming back to play the next day.

How is a bad shot, I now wondered for the first time in my life, *any different than losing control of my bowels?*

I knew I could hit ten or fifteen bad shots and *still* end the round with a respectable score of eighty-five. So was it conceivable that I could crap my pants on the bus, right in front of everybody, and *still* go on to have a pretty good day? Until right then, I'd never even considered the possibility that having a public accident was something a person could recover from.

And if that *was* true, then did it make any sense to keep avoiding activities I was too scared to do just because my bowels might hit a bad shot?

I certainly didn't think any less of Bam—as a golfer or as a person—just because he'd hit that horrible shot. He'd cost us the match, and in my eyes, Bam was still very much the man.

Maybe he wouldn't have thought any less of me if I had soiled my khakis on the bus. But then again, maybe I was trying to stretch Teddy's wisdom too far.

◆   ◆   ◆

In our room the next morning, Bam asked me if I'd been sick. He'd heard the toilet flush several times during the night.

"Yeah, sorry about that," I said. "That dinner really did a number on me. I hope I didn't wake you."

He smiled. "Don't worry. If anyone understands what it's like to have gastrointestinal problems, I do."

"How so?"

"My doctor diagnosed me with something called IBS," Bam said in a surprisingly matter-of-fact manner. "It stands for irritable bowel syndrome."

I just stood there, mouth open, speechless. I never would have suspected that Bam, of all people, had IBS. After a few seconds, I managed to nod and utter, "Really?"

"Yeah, apparently it's pretty common," he said.

I still couldn't get over how forthcoming he was. He was talking about his IBS as if it were no big deal, as if he had high blood pressure or tendonitis.

He was also the first person I'd ever met who'd been officially diagnosed. I had so many questions. Where to start?

"So do you have to watch what you eat?" I asked.

"Not so much," he said. "My doctor said that, for me, stress is what sets off my symptoms. I don't know if you've noticed, but I can get pretty wound up."

"It doesn't seem to affect your golf game," I said, assuming his earlier outburst had been the byproduct of nothing more serious than a bad temper.

"Oh, yeah? Check this out: a few years ago I was playing in a big tournament. We were on the eighth hole, and I was leading the field by three strokes. All of a sudden, my bowels started going nuts. I knew the closest bathroom was still three holes away, so I started to get really nervous. I didn't think I'd be able to make it."

"So what happened? Did you make it?"

"No," Bam said. "I ended up losing it right there on the course, right in front of everybody. Want to know the worst part?"

I nodded. What could possibly be any worse?

"I was wearing *white* pants."

"Oh my God! How did you finish the tournament?"

Bam shook his head. "I didn't. I forfeited and got the hell out of there as fast as I could."

"Whoa, that must have sucked. Has it gotten any better since then?"

"The doctor put me on some medication. It helps me calm down and keeps me from getting so stressed out. It seems to be working."

"The reason I'm so curious is because I'm pretty sure I have IBS, too," I said, "although I've never talked to my doctor about it."

"You should," Bam said. "You *definitely* should."

◆   ◆   ◆

"I was beginning to wonder if you were ever going to come," Johnny said, as he gave me a hug and helped me lug my bags into his apartment. "So, how was Ireland?"

Johnny was my mother's cousin. But since neither of us was sure exactly where that left us, we'd always referred to ourselves as cousins, too. He'd been living overseas for almost twenty years, so we only saw each other sporadically, mostly at weddings and funerals every couple of years. He would always throw out the same open-ended invitation: "Anytime you want to come for a visit, you've got a free place to stay."

To which I would always respond, "This year I'm going to try to get over there. I promise. Really."

To which my mother would say, "Tim, I'm telling you. If you don't take him up on his offer, you're *insane*. I honestly don't know what you're waiting for."

After a quick celebratory glass of champagne, Johnny couldn't wait to show me around. It was a warm, sunny Sunday afternoon. "Feel like going for a walk?"

"I'd love to," I said. I could feel my heart beating faster.

It felt just like the pent-up anticipation in those final few seconds before losing my virginity to Emily Becker in the woods in tenth grade. I knew what was about to happen, yet I had no idea what it was going to *really* feel like. After years of yearning and fantasizing, would it live up to my expectations? Could it possibly be even better than I'd imagined?

Walking down the staircase, I got the chills.

I stepped out that door and onto the street, knowing I'd never be the same person again. I'd never get another first time. The cab ride from the airport didn't count. Looking out the windows had been titillating, but it still felt like watching a movie. It wasn't real enough.

From Johnny's apartment, we meandered our way up one curving cobblestone road after another. We were walking uphill, but the grade was so gradual and our pace was so leisurely, it was hard to notice.

Locals and tourists filled the streets and the cafés. Around each twisting turn, I found another new picturesque tableau—new architecture, new women, new restaurants (with bathrooms, I assumed)—that I got to see for the very first time.

Someday people would ask me what it was like. I wanted to take it all in, every last detail, so I would never forget *exactly* what it felt like. But that was difficult because I still felt like I was in a dream.

The road leveled off, and we turned one last corner. To our left, an enormous cathedral leaped from the ground. To our right, in front of the cathedral, was the top of a set of stone steps. I followed my cousin over to the top of the steps.

"Well, what do you think?" Johnny asked.

What I saw caught me completely by surprise. Sure, I'd seen this exact view, and hundreds just like it, in my textbooks and on TV. But this was different. This was so much better.

Hundreds of feet below our position at the top of Montmartre, spread out like a painting, the city of Paris was laid out in front of me: La Seine, Le Louvre, Notre Dame, L'Arc de Triomphe, Le Jardin des Tuilleries, Le Champs-Elysees … and, of course, La Tour Eiffel.

What did I think?

"*Whoa!*"

I couldn't wait to get down there and take a closer look.

◆   ◆   ◆

It was two thirty in the afternoon. My feet were tired, and I was hungry and thirsty. It was time to take a break.

By day I was a tourist, which suited me just fine because I had plenty to do.

Each morning, after Johnny left for the office, I loaded up my little backpack with everything I might need for ten hours of exploring the Paris streets and walked out the door.

In front of the futuristic Pompidou Center, I found a café and plunked myself down at one of the outdoor tables.

The waiter came over and, in perfect English, asked me, "Yes, what would you like today?" He didn't even *try* to ask me in French. I guess the mountain of postcards I'd pulled from my backpack marked me as a tourist.

Nonetheless, I asked him, *en français*, for a Croque Monsieur sandwich and a glass of Bordeaux, "s'il vous plait."

"Trés bien, monsieur," he said with a smile. "Merci beaucoup."

It was the simplest, most mundane exchange of information. But, to me anyway, it was thrilling to be understood.

Now I wanted to make everyone back home understand me. I wanted them to see that I'd become a new person. I grabbed my pen and reached for the postcards.

Dear Mom,

Paris is INCREDIBLE! I've only been here a couple of days, but I've already been to the Eiffel Tower, Notre Dame, and the Louvre. I speak French every chance I get, and people actually understand what I'm saying ... most of the time, anyway. Johnny is throwing a small dinner party tonight, so I'll get to practice even more with his friends. I wish I could stay here for another month.

Love, Tim

P.S. How come you never took me to Paris?

My seat at the café was turning out to be a fantastic spot for people watching, so I decided to stay put for a while. Like the other seventy or eighty people sitting around me, I was perfectly content to sit back, sip a glass of wine, and watch the world pass by.

I looked over at my backpack. For three days, I'd been lugging around the added weight of an extra pair of jeans and a Gore-Tex pullover that I could quickly wrap around my waist. I preferred to think of it as an insurance policy of sorts, but there was no getting around what it really was: my security blanket.

Only now did it dawn on me that, so far, I'd been carrying all this extra clothing around for no good reason. Why, I wondered, had my bowels been so well behaved since I got there, even when I rode the Metro?

With a comfortable seat at the café, I had all afternoon to think about it.

Part of the answer seemed obvious: I was on vacation. In Paris my time was my own. Unlike in Ireland, I didn't have to be on a bus at a certain time. I didn't have to adhere to anybody else's schedule. I could stop and use a restroom anytime I felt like it without feeling like I was putting anybody out. Except for Johnny, *nobody* knew me in Paris, which meant nobody had any expectations of me, either. I could be as anonymous as I wanted to be.

But my invisibility didn't explain everything. There had to be more to it than that.

Three hours and three glasses of Bordeaux later, I figured it out. It was right in front of me.

Like any major metropolitan city, Paris had a distinct energy. But despite traffic jams and crowded shops, the energy in Paris was not the frenetic pulse you would find in New York, LA, or San Francisco.

The city just had a different feel to it. The absence of tension in the air was palpable.

Nobody seemed to be in a hurry to do anything. Parisians, even ones with "full-time" jobs, still managed to find time in the middle of the day to sit down at an outdoor café, have a beer or a glass of wine, smoke a cigarette or ten, and simply enjoy life.

Later that night, over a few glasses of cognac, I told Johnny how much I'd enjoyed Paris and appreciated his hospitality.

"Why don't you stay a little longer?" he asked. "It would be great if you could at least stay through the weekend."

"Believe me, if I could, I'd love to stay here for a few more months."

"So what's stopping you?" Johnny asked. Spoken like a true Parisian.

"Are you kidding? After seven days in Ireland and five days here, I'm already pushing my luck. Besides, I've got to leave for a big business trip to St. Louis on Monday. If I'm not back in time, I don't think I'll have a job to go back to."

"That's too bad," Johnny said.

"Yeah, tell me about it."

Now that I'd tasted the good life, I wasn't so sure I wanted to return to my backyard. Maybe Bowie wasn't so dumb after all.

I reminded myself it wouldn't be that bad. After all, I was going back to another picturesque city, a stylish apartment, and a prestigious career that paid me a handsome salary. Now that my passport was broken in, and my confidence was soaring, I'd be going back to San Francisco a far more eligible bachelor.

Fight or Flight

Everybody gave me the same advice. They repeated it, one after another, like a mantra: "Get on a plane. Take a vacation. That's what I'd do."

The problem, of course, was that I'd just gotten back from vacation. I'd only been home three days. Packing my suitcase and flying out again was the last thing I felt like doing. In hindsight I should have stayed in Paris.

Would it have been so hard to send me a fax? How about a phone call? Hell, I would have settled for an e-mail. I'd burned up one hundred thousand hard-won frequent-flier miles for that trip. Seriously, somebody really should have found a way to give me the news before I got back on that plane.

But no, that wasn't the way it had gone down. Paul had decided to wait until I was back in San Francisco, and on my way to catch my flight to St. Louis, to tell me I had been fired.

To justify my termination, Paul—accurately—cited my "propensity for canceling sales meetings." Also mentioned was my absolute unwillingness to hop on a plane and fly to the middle of nowhere so I could "run out the ground ball" on leads I was quick to label "real long shots."

"You're just not putting in the effort," he'd said.

I can't say it had come as a complete surprise. I often wondered how I'd managed to last as long as I had.

I spent most of September holed up in my apartment, adrift in a sea of self-doubt and introspection, trying to come to grips with my

211

professional future and where this development left my value on the San Francisco dating market. Becoming an international traveler was all well and good, but now that I lacked both a career *and* a set of reliable bowels, I was bracing myself for a long dry spell.

Around the end of the month, Steve called. "Hey, Tim, I've got an extra ticket to a charity party tonight. I know you're not a big fan of black-tie events, but I've heard there are going to be a ton of single women there. Want to join me?"

Even though it had been a rough month, and I was expecting things to get worse, I had to get out of my apartment, throw back a few drinks, and let loose.

"Sure, why not?" I said, searching my closet for my clip-on bow tie.

When we walked into the party, Steve could hardly contain himself. Beautiful women were everywhere—hundreds of them, wall to wall. Fish in a barrel, as the saying went.

But this would be one night when Steve and I wouldn't have to worry about competing for the same women. In my battered state, I had no expectations whatsoever. My plan was to hang out at the bar and not even look at them. Besides, I was woefully unprepared to tackle the cornerstone question of small talk, "So, what do you do?"

While Steve worked the room, I stayed put at the bar. Three margaritas and two shots of Jägermeister later, I was shocked to find myself on the receiving end of a series of flirtatious smiles. *Is she looking at me? No way, she can't be.* After our eyes met a half dozen times, she walked over from the dance floor.

"I'm Elizabeth," she said with a slight Southern accent. So simple. So bold.

"Hi, Elizabeth. I'm Tim. Can I interest you in a margarita?"

Let the small talk begin.

Unlike me, Elizabeth had a career—a good one, too. The way she described it, the perks of her marketing job nearly qualified her to be profiled by Robin Leach on *Lifestyles of the Rich and Famous*: a brand-new BMW convertible, an unlimited expense account, reservations at the city's hottest five-star restaurants, and season tickets to the symphony.

She didn't need to post her picture on Match.com. Each week, thanks to the high-profile charity events her company sponsored, Elizabeth's smiling face was splashed all over San Francisco's society pages. If ever somebody loved her job, it was Elizabeth.

"So, Tim, what do *you* do for a living?"

With no expectations to begin with, I had nothing to lose. Why not put a humorous spin on my predicament? It wasn't as if this conversation were going to last more than a few minutes anyway.

"Well, I used to work in the investment business," I said, confirming I'd once been respectably employed. "But now I'm enjoying temporary early retirement."

Technically this was true. I hadn't started looking for a new job yet, choosing instead to subsist on my small severance package and the modest savings I had squirreled away.

To my surprise, Elizabeth smiled. She probably thought I was one of those dot-com millionaires who had the luxury of not working anymore.

As we talked and drank through the night, we discovered we belonged to the same gym, lived in adjacent neighborhoods, and grew up on the East Coast. San Francisco was a small city where everybody seemed to know everybody—and date them, too. How was it possible we'd never met?

As it turned out, the closest Elizabeth and I had ever come to running in the same circles was on the treadmill at the Bay Club. But even then, she worked out at dawn, while I preferred dusk. The fact of the matter was that we led very different lives that were unlikely to ever intersect. I didn't hang out much at the symphony, and she'd never be caught dead in a place like Café Marimba. She may not have been the type of woman I ordinarily would have dated, but since I wasn't expecting much in the way of other options, I didn't see the harm in opening myself up to new experiences.

◆   ◆   ◆

Four months later, new experiences were exactly what Elizabeth and I were discussing over lunch.

Her eyes lit up, and she could hardly contain herself.

"Listen to this. I'm thinking about going to Vienna and Budapest for my vacation this spring, and maybe even checking out Prague while I'm over there. Doesn't that sound great?"

Vienna … Budapest … Prague … My first reaction was visceral. I looked around the restaurant to locate the men's room.

My relatively short history with this woman had taught me this was no time to voice such candid thoughts. It didn't happen often, but she'd been known to take great personal offense with what I considered an innocuous difference of opinion. "Yes, I would like butter on the popcorn," had been one of my more memorable infractions.

Were these nasty rebukes a sign of incompatibility? We had only been dating for four months, too soon for either of us to know how things would work out. Nevertheless I still tried to avoid such outbursts at all costs.

The trip to Ireland and Paris, though a breakthrough, hadn't obliterated my old thought patterns and physical reactions. My Invisible Fence had lost much of its power, but it took a few seconds for my conscious brain to catch up with my gut. When it did, I was able to process Elizabeth's question more rationally.

Hey, new places are always frightening. But where is Vienna? It's in Europe. And you've been to Europe, remember? Budapest and Prague are right next door. So what's the big deal? This is nothing to get worked up over, right? Right.

"That does sound like a cool vacation," I said, trying to match her enthusiasm. "How did you come up those cities?"

She explained this trip was one of the perks of working in marketing. A local TV station had put this luxury vacation together, extending invitations to its best clients as a token of appreciation for their past—and future—business.

"That sounds like a great way for them to thank their clients," I said.

"No, I don't think you understand how big of a deal this is," Elizabeth said. "They don't invite just *anybody* on these trips."

"No?"

"No, you have to be pretty high up, pretty important. Usually only senior-level executives and their spouses are asked to go. I've been waiting years for one of these invitations."

She exuded the aura of someone whose undeniable value to the world had finally been recognized. Like Navin Johnson in *The Jerk* after he discovered his name in the phone book, Elizabeth was now *somebody*.

Since her response to my next question was bound to offer a hint as to where she saw us heading romantically, I decided to push the issue. "Who are you going to take?"

It was an awkward question that I wasn't sure I wanted to have answered—especially if the answer wasn't, "Well … you, of course."

She told me she had asked her younger sister to tag along, but had since rescinded the offer after not hearing back from her after two days. "She had her chance."

I decided to push the issue a little further.

I asked, "You didn't want to invite me?"

"Of course I did, sweetie, but I didn't think you would be able to go," she said. "You know … long flight … foreign countries … your whole IBS problem. I thought the whole trip would freak you out, so I didn't even bother to ask. Was I wrong?"

Was she wrong? Or did she have me pegged? I needed more time before I said anything I'd later regret. I stuffed the remainder of my burger into my mouth and raised my index finger to let her know I'd have an answer for her shortly.

When I'd *finally* gone to see Dr. Olson two months earlier, he diagnosed me with IBS and gave me a prescription for a low dose of Paxil. Calming my mind, he'd said, would help calm my digestive tract and help break the cycle. So far I hadn't noticed much improvement, but I wasn't going to let *that* stop me from going back to Europe.

"Do you *want* to go?" Elizabeth asked, filling the silence and implying the spot was still available. It wasn't as much of a question as it was a challenge. She was basically saying, "Let's see what you're made of."

With all the outward confidence I could muster, I blurted out, "Yes, I'd love to go."

"Are you sure?"

"Why are you so surprised? I think you're forgetting something here. I've already been to Paris and Ireland. Why would you think I couldn't do this?" I'd left out the part about the Drain-then-Seal technique.

"All right," she said, "but once you commit, there's *no* getting out of it. If we're not dating each other in two months, you *still* have to go. These tickets aren't transferable. Agreed?"

"Yes," I said, "it's a deal."

A week later, when she e-mailed me the itinerary, I came to a set of sobering conclusions: I was in way over my head; and I needed some serious help if I had any shot of pulling this off.

When I tried to back out, Elizabeth said, "If you ever want me to speak to you again, you're getting on that plane."

◆   ◆   ◆

Looking up at the building, I did a double take. *This can't be right.*

I looked down at the business card in my hand. Sure enough, I was exactly where I was supposed to be. The last time I had walked into this building, my boss, Paul, had told me to pack my personal items and never return. How ironic that the help that might have saved my career had been so close by all this time.

The last thing I needed was to run into any of my former colleagues. "Oh, I've got an appointment with a therapist. Yeah, she's going to try to rewire my thoughts so I can vacation in Europe without my bowels going into a complete panic attack every time I stray more than a hundred yards from a toilet." That would make for one unforgettable elevator ride.

Before setting foot into the lobby to commence my covert operation, I had already committed to my cover story du jour: "I'm stopping in to say hi to an old family friend. She works up on the sixth floor … some kind of shrink or something, I think."

This appointment had been Dr. Olson's idea. After the antidepressants didn't do the trick, he thought I should explore cognitive-behavioral therapy as a way to treat the anxiety that he believed was responsible for triggering—not causing—my IBS symptoms.

A polished brass plate was attached to the door: Suite 620, Heather Wassarman, PhD. I turned the handle and walked in to find an empty waiting room. Taking quick inventory, I was relieved to see I had everything I needed to make my wait an enjoyable one: two black, plastic chairs; a coffee table topped with recent copies of *Newsweek* and *People*; a four-foot-high electric waterfall kind of thing; and best of all, hanging prominently on the wall next to the door, his and hers restroom keys—mine for the taking. If the rest of the world were as accommodating as this tiny, sparsely decorated waiting room, then I would have had no need to spend even five seconds in this tiny, sparsely decorated waiting room.

I had barely gotten through the *People* table of contents when Dr. Wassarman opened her office door. She introduced herself with a handshake and a warm smile that immediately put me at ease. "Please, come in and have a seat," she said.

She sat down, opened a manila folder, and clicked her retractable pen. "We talked on the phone a little bit about your condition. If it's OK with you, I'd like to start by having you explain how IBS affects your daily life, what situations tend to trigger your symptoms, and why you're seeking treatment now."

"Sure, that's fine," I said. "Can I start with the last question?"

She nodded. "Whatever you want to do is fine with me."

"In six weeks, I'm going to Europe with a girl I've been dating, and I need to overcome my IBS before I leave. That's why I'm here."

The words *overcome my IBS* sounded ridiculously bold as they left my mouth. I didn't want to get my hopes too high. I was skeptical, but I desperately wanted to believe this could work.

"OK, to help me understand this, what would happen if you went on this trip without any improvement to your condition?" she asked.

"Oh, my God, it would be a disaster," I said. "I've gotten to the point where I'm obsessed with always knowing the exact location of the nearest toilet. Whenever I don't know where the bathroom is, or whenever I'm trapped and I know I can't easily get to one, that's when I start freaking out. I avoid these situations every chance I get."

"Can you give me some examples of these situations?"

"Sure. How much time do you have? Well, for starters, there's getting stuck in traffic when I'm riding with other people, being trapped in my seat on a plane whenever the seat belt sign is on, and going to the dentist or the barber. Sitting anywhere but in an aisle seat is completely out of the question."

"I see. So what you're saying—"

"But that's just scratching the surface. I refuse to go to plays and the symphony, too. My mother thinks I'm an atheist because I won't go to church with her. To round out the short list, I would add waiting in the airport security line and riding on planes or buses that don't have restrooms. How's that for an answer?"

Dr. Wassarman was frantically scribbling to record my litany of phobias.

After catching up, she asked, "What exactly do you fear about them?"

"I'm scared I'm not going to be able to get to a bathroom before I have an accident," I said, then added for clarification, "you know, crap my pants. It's bad enough if it happens when I'm alone, but the thought of being humiliated in front of an audience, like on a plane or a bus, really makes me freak out. What would people do? What would they think of me?"

Dr. Wassarman looked up from her notes. "That's the second time you've used the term 'freak out.' Are you saying your head fills up with catastrophic images?"

"Well, yeah, but that's only part of it. At the same time my mind fills up with worst-case scenarios, my digestive tract does everything it can to empty itself as quickly as possible. The panic might start in my mind, but it moves instantly to my colon. Once the process starts, I have to find a bathroom right away. I know it sounds crazy, but that's what happens."

"No, it's not crazy. What happens in your mind can affect your body, and what happens in your body can affect your mind," she said. "You're describing what's known as the brain-gut connection."

"Yeah, well, I think in my case, a more accurate name would be the brain-*butt* connection."

"OK, let's get back to your trip to Europe," she said. "What particular aspects are causing you to freak out?"

Talk about a loaded question. The answer was at once so obvious to me and yet so difficult to articulate. It was like being asked, "What particular aspects of being mauled by a pack of grizzly bears do you find frightening?" The only honest response was, "I hadn't really thought about it like that, but now that you ask, absolutely everything."

I realized if she was going to be able to help me, I would have to itemize my fears.

"In the big picture, I'm freaking out because I know I'm not going to have any control over any aspect of this trip," I said. "Somebody else is running the show, and I will be completely at their mercy." I explained how all the meals, flights, trains, buses, sightseeing trips, and evening entertainment had all been planned to the minute. Every hour of every day, I would have no choice but to be in a specific place at a specific time. There was no wiggle room in the itinerary. I added, "What if I suddenly have to go to the bathroom?"

"That's a good question," she said. "What do you think would happen if you had to go at an inconvenient time?"

"I'd only have two choices, and they're both terrible. I could try to find a restroom—which would throw everybody off schedule—or I could relieve myself on the spot and ruin the event for all those unlucky enough to be within sniffing distance. Either choice would draw unwanted attention. I feel so much pressure not to screw up and let everybody down."

"Who is *everybody*?" Dr. Wassarman asked.

"Elizabeth and I are one of forty or fifty couples going on this trip. So from the second we get on the plane in San Francisco until we get back eight days later, I'll have a constant audience of close to a hundred people. Let's say I have an accident on the flight *to* Europe. It's not like I'm never going to see these people again. I'm going to have to eat every meal with them, sit next to them on the bus, socialize with them over cocktails, and then fly back to California with them. What's worse is they all have business ties with Elizabeth. So if I mess up, it's going to make her look bad, too."

"Let's talk about Elizabeth for a minute," Dr. Wassarman said. "How does she feel about your IBS? Is she supportive?"

This was another good question. To the degree that Elizabeth had not stopped dating me after I'd confided my secret to her, yes, she was supportive. If it implied a genuine concern for my well-being and a willingness to go out of her way to accommodate my condition ... then, well, not so much.

"More or less," I said. "She's not bothered that I have IBS, but she's told me more than once that she thinks it's all in my head, and that it's not really a medical problem. So, when I start panicking about finding a bathroom, she gets annoyed and acts like she's the one being inconvenienced."

"Hmmmm," Dr. Wassarman said. "That's interesting. Would you say her attitude is making this trip more stressful for you?"

"Absolutely," I said. "It adds a ton of pressure."

"Let me ask you a blunt question. If this vacation is causing you so much anxiety, why do you want to go?"

This question didn't require any additional thought. It wasn't so much that I was fighting for a future with Elizabeth—who knew where we were headed? I was fighting for the chance to turn the tide, take charge, and live a normal life for the first time since reaching legal drinking age. Put into the clichéd, post-9/11 terminology, if I didn't go on this trip to Vienna and Budapest, my bowels would win.

"I'm going because I'm sick and tired of living such a restricted life."

She smiled, then lowered her head to make another notation in the manila folder.

"Let me explain how this works," Dr. Wassarman said. "Cognitive-behavioral therapy is based on the idea that our thoughts, assumptions, and beliefs determine how we react to external events. People with anxiety disorders or phobias have what we call cognitive distortions, or irrational thinking patterns, which give them a distorted view of what's really happening to them—and for no good reason."

She said that, left unchecked, these automatic, negative thoughts could race through my head and take me from a state of calm to an all-out, fight-or-flight response in no time—even when there was no real threat. She called this process *catastrophizing*.

"I want to make sure I understand this," I said. "By thinking people are going to laugh at me, or even beat me up, if I get up in the middle of a play to use the restroom, I'm catastrophizing?"

"Yes, that's a perfect example of a cognitive distortion," she said. "So the good news is that by changing the way you think, you can change the way you react to an event like that."

"That's all there is to it?" I asked.

"Well, not exactly," Dr. Wassarman said. "As you learn these new, or more adaptive, thoughts, you're going to practice them by exposing yourself to all the real-life situations that trigger your symptoms. Because cognitive-behavioral therapy focuses not just on distorted thoughts, but also on the feelings of anxiety and avoidance behavior, these exposure sessions are going to decrease your fear by decreasing your avoidance of anxiety-provoking situations. It is hard work, but eventually you're going to notice your fears will start to lose their destructive power over you."

"That sounds good to me," I said. "Let's get started."

"I think we have a good-sized list of triggers to work with. Since we only have six weeks, which ones should we focus on?"

I told her that even though I'd already flown to Europe without incident, the thought of sitting on the plane with Elizabeth and the other hundred guests was still a source of great anxiety. Even with the trip still so far away, I'd already lost sleep over taking a cab to the airport, sitting in the security line, and standing on the crowded jetway.

"You said you're going to be riding a lot of buses over there," she said. "Is that one you'd like to tackle before the trip?"

"No … that's a big one, but it can wait until I get back," I said. "Elizabeth said the buses all have bathrooms."

"Well, it's nice to have one less thing to worry about, isn't it?"

I smiled. "You can say that again."

In between my twice-weekly appointments with Dr. Wassarman, I had lots of homework to do.

I left each session armed with a list of fears to confront, an arsenal of deep-breathing exercises, a set of "coping cards" to remind me of my new thoughts, and a "Thought Record Sheet" to track my hourly anxiety level on a scale from one to ten.

I would spend the next six weeks purposely going to the movies and *not* sitting on the aisle, deliberately bothering people so I could use the bathroom, driving in rush-hour traffic after drinking my morning coffee, wandering for hours at a time through the international terminal at SFO, and even waiting in the airport security line.

If this didn't work, I had no idea how I was going to survive this vacation.

Luck Favors the Prepared

Elizabeth and I wheeled our bags out into the parking lot. After seventeen hours of traveling, I was ecstatic to see the two shiny luxury coaches waiting to whisk our group to our downtown hotel. Now I could really relax.

Dr. Wassarman would have been so proud.

Back in San Francisco, I'd breezed through the cab ride to SFO, the snaking airport security line, and even the slow, claustrophobic boarding process without the slightest protest from my digestive tract.

Even when Elizabeth and I had taken our seats, I'd felt no compulsion to visit the lavatory—truly unheard of. In fact, I had felt so well prepared, I couldn't wait for the seat belt sign to light up, so I could prove to myself—and Elizabeth—how far I'd come. When we finally did push back from the gate in San Francisco, it felt anticlimatic. *Why have I been so scared of this?* The rest of the eleven-hour flight to Frankfurt was a nonevent, as was the connecting flight to Vienna.

Yes, the money I'd paid Dr. Wassarman had been well worth it. All the trigger situations we'd focused on and practiced no longer produced the anxiety that set off my IBS. I couldn't wait to get back and finish tackling the rest of the triggers on my list.

Elizabeth and I handed our bags to the driver and stepped up into the bus. With the hardest part now behind me, the only thing left for me to do was enjoy five days of all-expense-paid sightseeing with a beautiful woman. That didn't seem too tough.

"What are you looking at?" Elizabeth asked.

"Nothing," I said.

"Then why do you keep looking at the back of the bus?"

"I'm trying to find the bathroom, but I don't see it."

Elizabeth turned around in her seat. "I don't see it, either. Oh, well. I'm sure it will be a quick drive to the hotel."

As our bus continued to fill up, I started fidgeting.

"Maybe the other bus has a bathroom," I said.

"Sweetie, you just went to the bathroom five minutes ago. Why would you possibly think you'd have to go again?"

"You don't understand. It doesn't work that way. You said there would be bathrooms on the buses. You were positive. Remember?"

"Well, I thought they would have them, but I guess they don't. There's nothing I can do about it, so you're just going to have to deal with it."

"*Deal with it?* How do you suggest I do that?"

"I don't know. You sure spent an awful lot of money with that therapist. She must have taught you *something.* Why don't you do some of your breathing exercises or pull out your little flash cards?"

"They're called coping cards, not flash cards."

"Whatever. Look, you told me you had a grip on your problem and could handle this trip. Now you're telling me you can't? How is that supposed to make me feel? This isn't just my vacation; it's also a business trip. So do whatever you have to do to deal with your problem, but just don't screw it up for me, OK?"

"Hey, I *did* get a grip on my problem, and you *know* I made a lot of progress. If you had told me the buses weren't going to have bathrooms, I could have practiced and prepared for this. But you said I wouldn't have to worry about this part of the trip."

All of a sudden I felt as if I were in one of those high-school nightmares where I walked into the SATs having studied only for the math section. *What do you mean there's a verbal section?*

For the first time in days, my anxiety level climbed past two. It was now hovering around four or five.

"It looks like we won't be leaving for a few more minutes," I said. "Maybe I can run back into the terminal. What do you think?"

The look on Elizabeth's face was not what I'd call supportive. "I cannot believe you're pulling this on me now. You're killing me. Hurry."

I got up from my seat just in time to hear the hydraulic doors hiss to a close and the bus's motor growl to life.

"Hello, my name is Gab-ree-*ella*," said a woman in broken English over the PA system. "It will be my pleasure to be your guide for the next five days in 'Veen' … yes, 'Veen' is spelled W-i-e-n and is German pronunciation for *Vee-enna*."

Looking out the window, I saw we had left the airport and were approaching a highway. I started in with my deep breathing. After inhaling long and slow until my diaphragm was distended enough to make me look eight months pregnant, I held my breath for one … two … three … four … five seconds and then … exhaled to release all my tension. *Again, inhale and hold for one … two … three … four … five seconds, and then … exhale …*

"We will be arriving in Veen at Hotel In-cont-in-*ental* within possibly forty-five minutes."

Hotel Incontinental? The guy across the aisle from us couldn't help but chuckle at that one. "God, I hope she meant *Inter*-continental."

"We do not know ex-*act* time because of maybe traffic in Veen, but you will be happy that I, Gab-ree-*ella*, will spend the time here with you to tell you all about the beautiful city of Veen."

I kept at the deep breathing, but it wasn't really doing the trick. I reached into my backpack and pulled out my trusty coping cards. Onto six white index cards, I'd written six new belief statements designed to help me put my fears into perspective. By focusing on these new beliefs, I would keep my irrational automatic thoughts at bay.

As I shuffled through the stack, I noticed they weren't all working quite as well as they had in the past.

"Even if the worst happens, it won't last forever."

That's true. Having an accident really wouldn't be the end of the world.

"It's OK to bother people when I need to use the bathroom."

Just make sure you don't bother Elizabeth.

"If I have an accident, most people will be sympathetic and understanding, not judgmental."

Yes, I believe most people will understand. Elizabeth, however, isn't most people.

"People are used to bad smells on airplanes."

Yeah, but I'm not so sure about buses.

"The odds of having an accident are slim. I've only had two public accidents in sixteen years."

That's a good point. The odds are heavily in my favor.

"No matter what happens, most people will still like me."

Again, I suspect Elizabeth is an exception.

The bus pulled off the highway and onto the city streets.

"To your left, you will see a *riv*-er. That, of course, is *Dan*-ube *Riv*-er. It is called Blue *Dan*-ube, but as you see, it is not blue at all. The *Riv*-er is quite, quite brown. But here in Veen, people still say 'beautiful blue *Dan*-ube.'"

As we sat in city traffic, I ripped through my coping cards again, repeating them over and over in my head. Elizabeth looked over at me, shook her head, and rolled her eyes.

"One thing the city of Veen is *fam*-ous for is *cof*-fee, very strong *cof*-fee. If you go walking from Hotel In-cont-in-*ental*, you will see many *cof*-fee houses. People like to sit and drink *cof*-fee all day and night at the *cof*-fee houses in Veen."

I set my coping cards on my lap and tried the deep breathing again, but Gabriella sure wasn't making things easy for me. *Strong coffee, brown river, and the Hotel Incontinental?* She knew all the right things to say.

Only with great effort was I able to wrestle my anxiety level from eight back down to four for the last fifteen minutes of the ride.

After we'd gotten to the hotel and checked in, Elizabeth and I took our bags up to our room. I opened the curtains and took in the aerial view of Stadtpark across the street.

Now that I'd survived my crisis on the bus, I was in a good mood again. "Pretty view, isn't it?"

"Yeah, it's beautiful," Elizabeth snapped. "Now shut the damn curtains, so I can get some sleep."

◆   ◆   ◆

The next morning, we ate breakfast in the lobby restaurant. With a good night's sleep under our belts, Elizabeth and I chalked up our bickering from the day before to being exhausted from the long trip. We each apologized and were back on good terms.

Our first order of the day was to choose between getting on a bus for a tour of the city and getting on a bus to drive to go see the Spanish Riding School.

Elizabeth read through the descriptions of each outing. "I've heard about the Lipizzaner Stallions they have at the Spanish Riding School. I think that would be really cool to see. What do you think, sweetie?"

"Yeah, I guess that sounds fine to me."

As I leaned in for another bite of my strudel, I saw two buses pull up and park in front of the hotel. *Are those our buses?*

"Excuse me," I said to Elizabeth. "I'll be right back."

A few minutes later, I came back to the table with a new plate and more strudel.

"You know," I said. "I think I'd rather tour the city than see the horses. What do you think about that?"

Elizabeth looked angry again. "What was all that about?"

"What was all *what* about?"

"Don't play dumb with me," she said. "I saw you talking to the bus drivers outside. What were you talking to them about?"

"Nothing, really."

"I don't believe you. I want you to tell me right now."

"All right, fine, I'll tell you. I asked them if those were our buses, and if they had bathrooms on them."

"I knew it," she said. "And what did they say?"

"They said all of the buses have bathrooms, even the one we took from the airport. Instead of being in the back, like they are in America, they're recessed into the side of the rear-door steps."

"See? You did all that worrying yesterday for nothing."

"Well, not really. Here's the thing. The drivers told me they only unlock the toilets for the trips that last more than an hour, like the city tour."

"So I can't go see the Spanish Riding School because you want to be on a bus with a bathroom?"

"I don't want to keep you from doing what you want to do," I said. "Go see the horses. I'm happy to see the city on my own. I don't mind."

I could see from Elizabeth's eyes she was about to explode.

"Are you kidding me? How do you think that's going to make me look if I get on that bus alone? People are going to think something's wrong between us. Nobody brings their spouse or significant other all the way to Europe only to do things separately."

"I'm sorry. I just don't feel comfortable getting on that other bus."

"Well, since you're obviously not giving me any choice in the matter," Elizabeth said, "I guess we should get moving."

Elizabeth waited in the restaurant while I went up to the room to gather my things. When I came back to the table, she took one look at me and rolled her eyes again. "You do know it's like ninety-five degrees outside, don't you?"

"Yeah, so?"

"So why are you wearing dark jeans?"

"Because I like them, and they're comfortable," I said. "What's the big deal?"

"I just don't understand why you'd want to sweat your ass off. And why are you bringing a backpack?"

"I want to bring my camera, my coping cards, and my notebook so I can write if I get a chance." I didn't tell her I'd also packed *another* pair of dark jeans and my Gore-Tex pullover.

"Oh, that reminds me. If anybody asks, don't tell them you're unemployed. You can say you're writing a book, but I'd rather you didn't say what it's about, OK?"

"Why not? I thought you didn't have a problem with it."

"I don't, but a lot of people might. I think it's great you finally feel comfortable enough to admit you have IBS, but I don't want you to go overboard."

"Overboard? What do you mean?"

"I mean you've been getting pretty evangelical about telling people lately. Not everybody wants to know you have irritable bowel syndrome. Trust me."

"So what should I tell them my book is about?"

"I don't know. Maybe you can say you're not at liberty to discuss it before it's published."

"Fine," I said. "Let's go get on the bus."

I knew I'd made the right choice when we made our first stop forty-five minutes later at a tourist attraction called—no kidding—the Toilet of Modern Art. Vienna was a city that had its priorities straight.

◆   ◆   ◆

Our third day in Vienna was hotter and more humid than the first two, and my dark jeans and backpack routine was wearing thin with Elizabeth.

"No, forget it. I'm not going to let you wear those jeans again. I know you packed a pair of nice shorts, so go put them on."

"Are you insane?" I said. "They're *khaki*!"

"You're going to be fine in khaki shorts … especially today. Come on, we've already been over this."

The whole group, all one hundred of us, would be traveling to Budapest aboard a restored Orient Express Pullman train that had been chartered just for us. Three hours later, we would step off the train and onto a waiting riverboat for an afternoon of food, wine, and sightseeing along the Danube. Elizabeth was right: aside from the quick bus ride to the train station, I couldn't ask for an easier bathroom day. Although I'd never admit it, I was way too hot in my jeans.

"OK, I'll wear the khaki shorts," I said, "but only if I can still bring my backpack."

"If that's what you think you need to do, then go ahead, I guess."

The train ride from Vienna to Budapest couldn't have been any more enjoyable. We got a chance to mingle and get to know the other guests much better. To Elizabeth's chagrin, I was pleasantly surprised to find out they were not at all the stuffy, pretentious snobs I'd been led to believe they would be. To the contrary: one guy owned and managed a couple of IHOPs in the Bay Area, and another handled the marketing duties for a local chain of auto parts stores. They were nice, friendly, down-to-earth people. While Elizabeth sat by herself and read her romance novel, I spent the whole ride chatting with them about everything except the subject of my book.

When the train pulled into Budapest, I grabbed my backpack and followed the crowd through the station. *How cool that we can hop off a train and then right onto a boat!*

I walked outside and didn't like what I saw. Not only was there no boat waiting, there wasn't even any water. No, all I saw was a concrete parking lot and two waiting buses. *Nobody said anything about a bus ride. Fuck!*

I turned around to run back into the station, but Elizabeth grabbed me by the arm. "Don't even think about it. We're getting on this bus with everybody else. Right now."

Looking down at my khaki shorts and realizing I had no idea how long we'd be on this bus, I clutched my backpack with a death grip. My anxiety level burst through six and began to accelerate. Still walking toward the bus, I closed my eyes and started the deep breathing exercises. *Inhale nice and deep, then hold for one ... two ... three ... four ... five seconds ... and now exhale ...*

I stepped up onto the bus and followed Elizabeth toward the back. Our seats were directly across from the bathroom door. *Hmmm … maybe it's unlocked. Wouldn't that be great?*

A woman walked by and pulled on the door handle. When it wouldn't open, she looked over at me. "Do you know if somebody's in here? I really have to go."

Elizabeth shot back, "No, it's locked."

I had to jump in and see if I could turn the situation to my advantage. "I'm sure the bus driver has a key. If you really have to go, why don't you go up and ask—"

Oooowwww! God damn it! Elizabeth's right elbow plowed into my left rib cage. "What the hell was *that* for?" I tried to whisper.

"Stop it, right now! You're embarrassing me."

OK, now it was time for the gloves to come off. *Screw Elizabeth.* She wasn't just refusing to help me; she was making things *worse* for me. I was going to have to tune her out and take care of myself. I pulled out my coping cards and struggled to wrestle my anxiety back down to a manageable level.

The bus ride to the river couldn't have taken any longer than ten minutes, but because I had no idea where we were going, it seemed to take forever. By the time we pulled up to the dock, Elizabeth wasn't speaking to me. That was OK, because I wasn't too interested in talking to her, either.

On the boat, we sat down for lunch in the glass-enclosed main cabin. When the server came by and set three bottles of white wine on the table, I reached over and poured myself a full glass. A minute later, I poured myself another. I might have been Elizabeth's guest, but this was my vacation, too, and I wasn't about to let her ruin any more of it for me. I was going to make the most of it and let the chips fall where they may.

As we cruised down the Danube toward the Chain Bridge, the other couples at our table thought it was a good idea to get to know each other a little bit. One by one, each person said a few words about themselves and answered whatever random questions the audience tossed their way.

"I'm Tim Phelan. I live in San Francisco, and I am Elizabeth's guest."

"Her *guest?* You're not married?" a man asked.

Elizabeth shook her head so hard I thought it was going to twist off. "No, we're not married."

"So, Tim Phelan from San Francisco, guest of Elizabeth, what do you do for work?"

Time for a little payback.

"I'm taking some time off from selling mutual funds so I can write a book."

"Really? What kind of a book?"

Elizabeth was giving me the death glare.

"It's a memoir," I said.

"About what?"

Elizabeth looked like she was about to explode.

"It's actually about living with a medical condition that's very common, but also very embarrassing."

"Now you've got me intrigued. You look perfectly healthy to me. What's the disease?"

I looked over at Elizabeth to let her know I held a few cards, too, and I was not afraid to play them. Her expression turned from furious to pleading. I'd made my point.

"I'd love to tell you, but I've probably said too much already," I said. "You'll just have to buy the book."

After lunch I walked out onto the deck and snapped some pictures of Budapest. I wanted to remember this part of the trip.

◆   ◆   ◆

By our fourth day in Europe, I was pretty sure Elizabeth wanted out of whatever was left of our relationship. I just underestimated how eager she was to expedite its demise.

"Since we have a free day tomorrow," she said, "what do you think about going to Prague?"

"Prague sounds cool. How long does it take to get there?"

"The concierge said we can make the trip in four hours."

"Four hours on a train doesn't sound so bad."

"No, it's four hours *by bus*," she said, her voice heavy with spite.

"Let me think about it."

I could see what she was up to. She figured suggesting a four-hour bus trip was just the way to draw me into a relationship-ending brawl, but this time she underestimated *me*. I didn't come all this way not to see Prague. On the way back up to our room, I stopped off to have my own chat with the hotel concierge.

"I talked to the concierge, and he said we could hire a private driver to take us to Prague and back. He'll even give us a tour of the city. What do you think?"

Elizabeth was caught by surprise. "And how much does that cost?"

"A couple hundred dollars," I said.

She was dying to shoot this plan down. "You don't expect me to pay for it, do you?"

"Nope. It's my treat."

When it was clear I wasn't letting her draw me into a fight, she sank even lower. "But you still don't have a job. How are you going to afford it? I still think we should take the bus."

Instead of taking the bait, I decided to kill her with kindness. "Don't worry about it. Since you were nice enough to invite me on this free trip, I figure this is the least I can do to show my gratitude."

"Fine, have it your way."

The next morning, we met our driver, Peter, outside and stepped into the back of his sedan. Before we even got on the road, Elizabeth made a big deal about my refusal to stow my backpack in the trunk as Peter had suggested.

"I think you wasted your time and money on all that therapy," she said. "If you can't even part with your backpack for a few hours, you obviously haven't made that much progress at all."

Elizabeth was right to point out that I hadn't exactly aced this test. Even I knew that. But for once I wasn't so ready to beat myself up for it. Neither of us had had any way of anticipating that the bus's bathrooms would be locked most of the time. Had I been given the chance to prepare for that kind of scenario, I was confident I would have handled it as flawlessly as I had handled the rest of the trip.

Elizabeth was wrong; I had made *a ton* of progress.

Because I no longer cared what she thought of me, I used the rest of our drive to practice something Dr. Wassarman had taught me: the belief that it's OK to bother people when I have to use the restroom.

Even though I didn't really have to go, I had Peter make no fewer than five pit stops on my behalf during the hour-and-a-half drive between the Czech border and Prague. I was delighted to find out Dr. Wassarman had been right. Peter didn't seem the least bit bothered by my frequent requests.

Despite the fact that she hadn't said a word to me since we'd left the Incontinental, I could tell I was pushing Elizabeth closer to her breaking point with each bathroom stop. A breakup was imminent.

Later that night, over dinner in Vienna, we made it official.

The long flight back to San Francisco gave me plenty of time to think about being single again. Maybe I'd meet somebody better down the road, or maybe I wouldn't … but I was prepared to take my chances.

Unfinished Business

"Well?" Dr. Wassarman asked with a polite smile.

Busted! Again.

I tried to look away. *No dice.* She wasn't about to let me off the hook.

"Do you have any particular news you'd like to share with me?"

I felt like a kid who was scared to tell his teacher he still hadn't completed the homework project he'd been assigned three weeks earlier—because I hadn't.

I looked at her and shook my head.

In the two months since I'd returned from Vienna a single man, I'd continued to see Dr. Wassarman each week. Under her tutelage, I had gained mastery over almost every trigger on our list. *Almost.*

I was hoping she would just forget about it. Why couldn't we spend the hour talking about my latest victories and call it a day? Wouldn't she rather hear about how I'd joined my friends for Sunday brunch on the other side of town, or how I'd told my dentist that my IBS might lead to an urgent bathroom trip?

But deep down, I knew she was right. My other triumphs were all well and good, but until I tackled this last assignment, I wouldn't feel the sense of accomplishment I craved so badly.

"I'll do it this week," I said.

My therapist lowered her glasses and looked me in the eye. "Do you promise?"

"Yes, I promise."

I wasn't just saying that, either. I was dead serious. Thanks to my looming assignment, my mornings spent at the Coffee Roastery on Chestnut Street had become bittersweet.

Oh sure, I cherished my newfound ability to sit by the front window in my khaki shorts while reading the paper and enjoying cup after cup of coffee without the slightest thought of humiliating myself. But my feeling of pride never lasted as long as I would have liked.

Every fifteen minutes, like clockwork, I was reminded of the work that remained to be done. Through the window I could only stare in fear as the giant beast strutted by, taunting me with its every step. It had been my nemesis ever since I'd moved to San Francisco in 1995—the #30 Marina Express bus, aka the 30X.

I'd tried to tell Dr. Wassarman that since I no longer worked downtown—or anywhere, for that matter—there was no real reason to make overcoming my fear of this bus a priority. While she had agreed I had no practical need to ride the 30X, she argued it would be a critical symbolic victory—especially after the bus fiasco in Vienna.

I knew she was right. The time had come for me to slay the dragon.

◆　　　◆　　　◆

As I locked my apartment door behind me, my anxiety level hovered around seven. I walked to the corner of Divisadero and North Point, two blocks from my house.

As I waited, about thirty kids poured out of the Marina Elementary School and began to run around the block for gym class. They were smiling, laughing, huffing, puffing, wheezing, and sweating. The scene got me reminiscing about my early years.

When I was their age, I remembered, I had been afraid of lots of things—tests, meeting new friends, having my lunch money stolen, and getting my ass kicked on the playground. To the best of my knowledge, however, boarding a bus and worrying about losing control of my bowels had never once crossed my mind. Those were the days.

Unlike the other yuppies waiting at the bus stop, I had no real reason to go to the Financial District. But I figured I might as well make the most of the trip, so I'd called my barber, Don, and scheduled a ten o'clock haircut.

I got on the bus, paid my $1.25 fare, and claimed a strategic seat up front. My anxiety level was creeping north of eight.

Two blocks later, we made our next stop. The bus was filling up quickly.

Time for some relaxation exercises. Let's get that anxiety level moving in the opposite direction.

Come on, pull yourself together and start the deep breathing … OK … inhale … one … two … three … four … five. Good, now hold the breath … one … two … three … four … five … Great, now exhale sloooowwwwlyyyy … one … two … three …

"Tim Phelan?"

I looked up and saw Sandra, a girl I had known growing up and now my neighbor again in San Francisco. We'd run into each other occasionally since I'd moved out west. Under any other circumstances, I would have been happy to see Sandra. Not today.

"What are *you* doing on the bus? Are you working again?" she asked, as she grabbed one of the few remaining seats, which just happened to be right next to me.

So much for my relaxation exercises.

"No. Not yet," I said. "I'm still on vacation."

I'd been hoping to carry out my experiment anonymously. After all, if things went awry, I sure didn't want anyone I knew to be a witness. I suppose it was an unrealistic expectation. San Francisco could be such a small city, where everybody seemed to know everybody. The Marina District was much smaller still. Sandra's arrival on the scene shot my anxiety level up to an eight.

"Actually, Tim, this is the first time I've taken the bus in years," said Sandra.

"Really? Me too," I said. *Just my luck.* Statistically I had a better chance of being struck by lightning. I made a mental note to buy a Lotto ticket on the way home.

Like all my other homework assignments, the idea behind this one was to gradually desensitize myself to the source of my anxiety. Dr. Wassarman had given me permission to attack this goal in small bites. On my first attempt, maybe I would ride the bus for only a few blocks. The next time, I would ride a few blocks more, eventually working my way up to a nonstop ride all the way downtown.

Because this was my first stab at this task, I had told myself I would take the 30X at least as far as the corner of Chestnut and Van Ness. That was the beginning of the express leg and the last chance to get on or off the bus until the driver opened the doors in front of the Transamerica Building on Montgomery Street. Secretly I was hoping to make it all the way.

When the bus rolled to its sixth stop, more well-groomed, pleasant-smelling, Stepford commuters piled in. To these throngs of Marina denizens, with their folded *Wall Street Journals* tucked under their arms and their laptop bags swinging from their shoulders, this was just another mundane morning commute.

"Hey, man, what's going on?"

I looked up and saw Kevin, an acquaintance I barely knew from the Bay Club. I gave him a nod as he walked toward the back.

Great! Now I've got two people who know me on this friggin' bus. Could it get any worse?

Yes, apparently it could.

When I looked around, it seemed as if the bus actually had pulled up to the bar at Cozmo's, the local meat market, and loaded up all the customers over the weekend. *So this is what they look like in the daylight. This town is way too small.* Riding the 30X was a lot like hanging out at Cozmo's, except for two differences: Cozmo's served drinks, and you could leave anytime you liked. On the 30X, you were sober and, for twenty minutes or so, you weren't going anywhere.

At the next three stops along Chestnut Street, no fewer than five more people I knew acknowledged me with a friendly "Hey, what's up?" or a flash of the eyebrows.

Will was a financial advisor I knew from the Marina deli. Kimberly was a woman I'd recently met at—where else?—Cozmo's. She'd given me her number a week or two earlier, but I hadn't called her yet. I also noticed two blondes whose names escaped me. I'd blown one off. The other had blown me off. So it goes.

Having my friends and neighbors on board was a double-edged sword. I felt comfortable around them—but not in this setting. It would be, I could only imagine, like running into a friend in a porn store. *Tim Phelan? Is that you? Hey, buddy, what's going on?* Find the nearest exit and get out of there.

Sandra said, "So I hear you're writing a book. What's that all about?"

"Oh, it's just something I'm playing around with—'funny stories that have happened to me' kind of thing. I think you'd get a kick out of it because a lot of it takes place in San Francisco."

"That sounds interesting. Am I in the book?"

"You are now."

Sandra and company were throwing off my game plan. With my anxiety spiking, my bowels growling, and my confidence slipping, I decided this would not be my day for a nonstop ride.

Peering through the sea of standing bodies clogging the aisle, I could see we were approaching Van Ness.

"Good seeing you, Sandra," I said. "This is where I get off."

She looked surprised. "You're getting off here? I assumed you were heading downtown."

"I am, but I have one stop to make here first."

"For what?"

For what? Good question. I have no idea.

"I promised a friend I'd feed his cat while he was out of town."

Feed my friend's cat? Guys don't have cats. Where did that come from?

Sandra smiled. "That's awfully nice of you."

"Yeah, what can I say? I'm sure he'd do the same for me."

"You have a cat?"

"No, I don't. But if I did, then I'm sure he would feed it. You know?"

"Uh-huh."

I reached up and yanked the cord to request a stop. When the doors opened, I squeezed through the bodies and bailed.

Slightly demoralized, but still determined, I decided I would hop aboard the next 30X that rolled along and resume my mission. Unfortunately the bus I'd just left turned out to be the last express of the morning. I would have to take the dreaded 30 Stockton.

The 30 Stockton was a local bus that wove its way through the Fisherman's Wharf area, North Beach, and Chinatown on its way to Union Square. In the Marina, it was known by the politically incorrect moniker of the Orient Express, which was a complete joke because nothing and nobody moved quickly through Chinatown. This bus stopped at least once on every block. A better name would be the "Slow Boat to Chinatown."

If I couldn't ride the 30X, I reasoned, I might as well ride *a* bus, even if it was the Slow Boat. Even though I knew I could get off whenever I wanted, maybe I could fool myself into thinking it was an express bus. It was worth a shot.

I paid another $1.25 and took another seat—I found plenty of empty ones. Several minutes later, that would no longer be the case. By the time we left Fisherman's Wharf, the bus was jam-packed with commuters and camera-toting tourists. I wasn't sure of the maximum number of passengers allowed on the bus by law, but it would be safe to say we were exceeding that limit by roughly—oh, I don't know—100 percent.

As our cattle car rolled toward North Beach, my nostrils inhaled the overwhelming stench of cheap cologne mixed with body odor. The pungent smell hung in the air like a blanket of San Francisco's thick morning fog. I relaxed when I realized having an accident on this bus would have the same effect as an air freshener. There would be no embarrassment and no shame.

When the Slow Boat finally pulled into Union Square, I disembarked and made my way toward the Financial District. I had the 10:00 AM appointment with my barber, and I didn't want to keep him waiting.

In the old days, I would spend the first five terrifying minutes in Don's barber chair concocting fictitious scenarios that would require me to shed my cape and run across the street. *Oh, no! Sorry, Don, but I think I left my wallet over at Starbucks. I'll be right back. I hope it's still there. I'd better hurry!*

But as I sat in the chair this time, I found it difficult to remember the panic I used to experience whenever I even thought about getting a haircut. This morning I'd walked directly from the bus to the Exchange Barber Shop without even entertaining the idea of ducking into the Bay Club across the street for a last-minute toilet trip. Thanks to doing my cognitive-behavioral homework, I was able to relax and listen to Don tell me about his upcoming family vacation to Disneyland.

So this is how normal people sit through a haircut.

Now, if I could only master the 30X …

◆　　　◆　　　◆

The next morning my alarm went off at 6:45.

After one cup of coffee, two pieces of toast, a shower, and a trip to the toilet (OK, three trips to the toilet), I was out the door and on my way. I was feeling optimistic but scared.

Since this was uncharted territory, and Dr. Wassarman had given me the green light to tackle this assignment in baby steps if necessary, I brought along my little backpack filled with most of the usual items: my coping cards; my blue Gore-Tex pullover; a pen and notebook (I wanted to record my anxiety level and also document the historic voyage); and my cell phone, just in case I needed to call a friend to pick me up.

As I walked to the bus stop, I reminded myself that the ride to Van Ness—the pre-express leg—should not be a source of any anxiety. This was the safest part of the expedition, and I had the confidence of having already made this part of the trip.

I'd decided the night before, barring any unforeseen change of events, that I would take a breather at Van Ness and break the trip into two segments. By getting an early start, I knew I could always shell out another $1.25 and hop onto the next 30X that rolled along.

The ride down Chestnut Street to Van Ness came along with the usual parade of friends, acquaintances, and Cozmo's regulars. But despite the audience of onlookers, the first leg of the trip was relatively free of anxiety. The desensitization was working. Spotting the intersection of Chestnut and Van Ness through the throngs of well-dressed straphangers, I tugged on the cord, squeezed past the beautiful people, and disembarked.

As I waited on the corner, I was all too aware that I was minutes away from coming face-to-face with my darkest remaining fear. Looking down the gentle slope of Chestnut Street, I could see my nemesis. The beast was still a half mile away, stopping on every block to fill itself to the gills with even more of my friends and neighbors. Pure evil.

Watching it plod toward me, I pulled out my coping cards and did some more deep breathing. No matter what I did, I couldn't get my anxiety level to dip below eight.

In an effort to make the unknown a little less unknown, I poked my head around the corner and surveyed the traffic on Van Ness, a major artery that was usually choked with commuters coming over the Golden Gate Bridge from Marin County.

The bus I had just left was stopped at the traffic light. *How long will it stay stopped?* I counted—exactly thirty-eight seconds.

About a hundred yards later, when the bus stopped at another light, I counted again—this time for fifteen seconds.

Once it cleared the second traffic light, the bus accelerated unimpeded toward the horizon. A little bit of quick arithmetic let me quantify my fear. It all came down to being able to survive for approximately fifty-three seconds. That still seemed like a long time, but it also seemed possible.

I was still terrified, but now at least I had a better sense of what to expect.

Looking down Chestnut Street, I could see it moving ever closer—now only one block away. *OK, Tim. It's time to find out what you're made of.*

I pulled five quarters from my pocket, took another deep breath, and stepped up to do battle.

I'd seen crowded buses before, but this was ridiculous. It was wall-to-wall bodies from back to front. The two men and one woman who got on just behind me collectively assumed the role of trash compactor, compressing me even farther into this hellish heap of humanity.

The driver closed the doors and, after a disconcerting five-second pause, made the right turn onto Van Ness.

Oh, God! There's no turning back now.

As I'd expected, we just missed the light at Van Ness and Lombard. While I waited for the light to turn green, I could feel my heart beating through my chest. I began to count to thirty-eight.

One … two … three … four … five …

My bowels were throwing their usual temper tantrum, but I kept counting. I had no other choice.

Seven … eight … nine … ten …

We must have been stopped right over the edge of my Invisible Fence. My insides were going crazy.

Don't listen to them, just keep counting. Twelve … thirteen … fourteen …

Just then, without any notice whatsoever, the bus lurched forward and picked up speed. *Hey, we're moving! What the …*

I'd only counted to fourteen. I had prepared myself for thirty-eight seconds at this light, and then another fifteen seconds at the next one. This wasn't how it was supposed to work.

Our stop at the second light was equally disappointing—only *six* seconds instead of fifteen. I'd paid good money for this challenge, and this was all I got?

Even though I had been scared to death just twenty seconds earlier, I now felt like I'd been cheated. And just like that, in the blink of an eye, my anxiety level plunged from ten to zero.

As the bus rolled through the Broadway tunnel and toward the Financial District, I couldn't conceal my grin. Cheated or not, I had done it!

I could feel people looking at me. *What's he so happy about?* I looked over my right shoulder at no one in particular. An attractive blonde entered my field of vision. She glanced up at me. I batted my eyebrows and shot her a confident grin. *Oh, yeah. I'm back!*

It reminded me of the summer I'd spent working up my courage to take my first ride on the terrifying Dragon Coaster at Playland. Once I'd realized it wasn't nearly as frightening as I'd made it out to be, I ran back through the line to ride it again and again.

I couldn't wait for my next appointment with Dr. Wassarman.

Epilogue:
A Regular Guy

Almost a year after my showdown with the 30X, I flew from San Francisco to Pennsylvania for my grandfather's funeral. After the viewing, my grandfather's five daughters, their current husbands, and most of his sixteen grandchildren all went to McCloskey's Pub across the street from the funeral home.

My cousin Jock, a perpetual wiseass, wanted an update. "So, Tim, what are you up to these days out in San Francisco? Did I hear your mom say you're writing a book or something?"

At that moment, all other conversations stopped. Everybody had heard Jock's question. *Writing a book?*

I tried to downplay the whole thing. "Yeah, it's nothing, really. It's actually more of a hobby than anything."

"What's it about?"

"I'd rather not get into it right now," I said. "Another time, I promise."

This just made the jackals lean in closer and start licking their chops.

"Oh, I don't think so," Jock said, taking the lead. "I think I speak for the entire family when I say we'd all like to know what you're writing about."

They'd all had plenty of alcohol and were starting to get a little belligerent. My cousin Johnny, from Paris, grabbed me by the neck and shook my head. "Tell us. *Now!* What is your book about?"

"Hey, all right. Fine, I'll tell you," I said. "Jesus. It's about IBS, OK?"

Now that he could smell red meat, Jock wasn't about to back off. He made sure to shout for maximum impact. "You don't mean *irritable* bowel *syndrome*, do you?"

Now everybody, including our waitress, was looking at me. This wasn't exactly the way I'd intended to tell my family what I'd been doing since I'd gotten fired, but I no longer had any choice. "Yes, that's exactly what I mean."

"Why are you writing a book about that?" my cousin Jim asked. "Do you *have* IBS?"

Thanks, Jock.

"Yup, I sure do," I said. "Or, I should say I *did*."

"You don't have it anymore?" my cousin Nina asked. "You're cured?"

I would have loved to say that my victorious ride on the 30X had turned out to be my last tango with my irritable bowels. Unfortunately, despite the dramatic progress I'd made, I'd be lying if I said I'd cured my IBS. That was just not the way it worked.

"Well, no, I still have occasional bad days here and there, but believe me, it's not *nearly* as bad as it used to be. There were so many things I wouldn't do for so many years because of it, but now I honestly feel like I've gotten my life back."

"How come I never knew about it?"

"It's not just you, Nina. Nobody did. It's not exactly the kind of thing you want to share with people, you know?"

Johnny's wheels were turning. "So, is that why you wouldn't come to Paris for all those years?"

I nodded. "You got it."

"Is that why you always drive by yourself?" Jock asked.

Again I nodded. "Uh-huh."

As we were leaving the pub, one of my aunts pulled me aside. "Listen, Timmy, I've had IBS for about ten years. It's horrible. Sometimes I can't even finish shopping at the grocery store. I'll be waiting in line, and then all of a sudden, I've got to get the hell out of there—and fast, you know?"

"Yup, I know."

The next morning, *another* one of my aunts confided that she'd had bouts of IBS throughout her adult life. She told me about the one time she was on a field trip with her daughter's class. As soon as the bus had pulled out of town, she had to beg the driver to pull over so she could knock on a total stranger's house and ask to use their toilet—which she did. "Do you have any idea how embarrassing that is?"

"Yup, I do."

At the reception after the funeral, I was approached by a *third* aunt. Missy—my so-called favorite aunt, the one who'd set me up with Kelly after college—asked me if I'd e-mail her some of the chapters I'd written. Why? She told me it was an issue close to her heart and had been for years. She shared stories of speeding down the Pennsylvania Turnpike at ninety miles per hour so she could get to the service area and use the bathroom.

Funerals have a way of bringing people together, but this was bizarre. I'd been living with IBS for sixteen years, and I'd had no idea that three of my aunts also had it. Crazier still, *they* didn't know it, either. Nobody talks about this stuff.

Once I started talking about my IBS, it was as if I discovered some secret society. Everyone I told about my condition either had it themselves or knew somebody who did. I know it's not the most pleasant conversational topic, but it seems ridiculous that our society can talk freely about erectile dysfunction, breast enlargement, gangster rap, and violence, but digestive disorders like IBS are off-limits. I wonder how many other people out there haven't gone for help because they're simply too embarrassed to even talk to their doctor about such a taboo topic.

Looking back, I realize my life didn't have to turn out the way it did. Those sixteen years after college could have been so much more fulfilling. How many great memories don't I have today because I let my embarrassment keep me penned up inside my Invisible Fence? I suppose it was better late than never, but my whole odyssey just seemed so unnecessary. What if I had gone to see a doctor right when I got my first symptoms after college?

On the positive side, I wouldn't be who I am today. For all the pain, angst, and lost opportunities, I'd like to think I learned an awful lot about myself in the process.

For starters, I'm more comfortable in my own skin, and I care much less about what other people think of me—even my mother. I learned the hard way that it's OK not to be perfect. It's OK to make mistakes. Life is a crap shoot, and accidents will happen. Once you accept these cold, hard facts, life gets a lot easier.

Also, in a strange way, IBS taught me about what's important to me. There's no doubt that listening to my gut deprived me of opportunities, but my gut wasn't wrong about everything. If it weren't for my cantankerous bowels, I might still be schlepping mutual funds today. Hell, I might have even ended up marrying someone like Elizabeth.

A few months after my grandfather's funeral, I told my mom I would be leaving San Francisco and moving back east with Heidi, my girlfriend of nearly two years. While she was ecstatic to hear the news, her joy was short lived. These days my mom is beside herself with angst because I still haven't walked down the aisle, and I continue to forgo a steady paycheck in favor of publishing my book.

It's not the idea of being a writer my mom objects to; she'd just prefer I write children's books instead of a memoir on irritable bowel syndrome. "My son, the IBS author" just doesn't have the same ring to it as "my son, the investment banker." Oh well, I know she'll still love me.

In one of the most fascinating experiences of my life, I drove from Philadelphia to Chapel Hill, North Carolina, to participate in an IBS research study. In an effort to determine the causes of IBS, the doctors at the University of North Carolina Center for Functional GI and Motility Disorders subjected hundreds of volunteers to a battery of tests that included a flexible sigmoidoscopy, hydrogen breath tests, blood tests, and even psychological questionnaires.

In layman's terms, here's what I took away from those two days as a guinea pig: The experts still aren't sure if IBS is one disease or many different diseases. Because no two people suffer from IBS in exactly the same way, it's not surprising that they all respond to different treatments in their own individual way. In other words, just because fiber and hypnosis didn't work miracles for my symptoms, that doesn't mean they won't do wonders for yours. Similarly, even though cognitive-behavioral therapy helped me get my life back, it might not be the answer for somebody else.

In a nutshell, one size does *not* fit all, and your actual mileage may vary. The most important thing is that people talk to their doctors about their symptoms *before* the condition takes over their lives.

One year after moving to Pennsylvania, Heidi and I went back to San Francisco for my buddy Mac's wedding. Walking through my old city, I didn't experience any of the same sensations of panic and rectal urgency that had been the hallmark of the decade I'd spent there. For old time's sake, I thought I'd treat Heidi to a pitcher of margaritas at Café Marimba. A notice on the locked door said it all: Café Marimba was no more.

No panic, no urgency, and now no Marimba? Had my time in this city all been a dream? Had any of it really happened? I shook my head, grabbed Heidi's hand, and strolled up Chestnut Street to see if Cozmo's was still around. Just then I looked up and saw a familiar sight. Rolling toward me was my old friend, the 30X. I couldn't help but smile.

Resources

To learn more about IBS, please contact the following organizations or visit their Web sites:

- **IFFGD, the International Foundation for Functional Gastrointestinal Disorders,** is a nonprofit organization that offers a wealth of reliable and useful information about IBS. They regularly publish information about IBS and related disorders contributed to them by an international group of medical experts. Find out more at this IFFGD Web site: www.aboutIBS.org or contact them at:

  IFFGD
  P.O. Box 170864
  Milwaukee, WI 53217
  Toll-free: 1-888-964-2001
  www.iffgd.org

- **The University of North Carolina Center for Functional GI and Motility Disorders** provides clinical care, research, health care professional training, and patient education in functional gastrointestinal and motility disorders.

  UNC Center for Functional GI and Motility Disorders
  UNC School of Medicine
  CB #7080, Bioinformatics Building
  Chapel Hill, NC 27599-7080
  (919) 966-0144
  www.med.unc.edu/ibs

- **The National Digestive Disease Information Clearinghouse (NDDIC)** provides information about digestive diseases to people with digestive disorders and to their families, health care professionals, and the public.

  National Digestive Disease Information Clearinghouse
  2 Information Way
  Bethesda, MD 20892-3570
  1-800-891-5389
  www.digestive.niddk.nih.gov/

- **The IBS Self Help and Support Group** is a patient advocate group in support of those who suffer from IBS, those who are looking for support for someone who has IBS, and medical professionals who want to learn more about IBS. The IBS Self Help and Support Group is the largest online community for people with irritable bowel syndrome. Visit their Web site at www.ibsgroup.org.

Acknowledgments

To say that I had help bringing this book into existence would be a colossal understatement. I owe a huge debt of gratitude to the following people:

Jim Mohan not only gave me the idea to turn my raw journal rants into a manuscript, but, years later, he also designed the book's cover. Over long, overpriced lunches at the Grove, Ed Waingortin gave me invaluable moral support to push ahead with this project when I was often tempted to walk away. Of course, I now feel compelled to thank John Rodakis, who, in addition to offering sound marketing advice, first introduced me to the aforementioned, indispensable Ed Waingortin.

John Distelhurst, my long lost friend from my middle-school days in Hastings, spent hours generously reading and rereading my early drafts and critiquing them with his refreshing, trademark bluntness. My cousin Ty DeCordova was a great sounding board, graciously spending the better part of two years listening to the ups and downs of this unusual project.

Jon Stenzler opened my eyes to the importance of hiring a professional editor. In addition to sharing his editing expertise with me, David Lee Preston became a friend and turned me into a far better writer than I ever would have become on my own.

I want to thank Dr. Heather Wassarman for helping me accurately describe the technical aspects of cognitive-behavioral therapy, and especially for making the last three chapters possible (for those of you who might want to work with Dr. Wassarman, she can be reached through her Web site at www.heatherwassarman.com).

Thank you to all my friends, bosses, co-workers, dates, girlfriends, and acquaintances who, even though your names have been changed, have become a part of this book. And to those who bravely declined the cover of an alias (especially Erin and Missy), I am enormously grateful.

I also want to thank all the writers and reviewers at Fanstory.com whose encouragement and constructive criticism gave me the confidence to take the final plunge into publishing this story.

Thank you, Heidi, for your love, your acceptance, and your endless patience.

And of course, I want to thank my family—Mom, John, Fred, Lisa, Melissa, Caroline, Emma, and Griffin—for all their support along the way.

978-1-58348-018-2
1-58348-018-8

30171012R00149

Made in the USA
Middletown, DE
23 December 2018